SATVIC MOVEMENT

THE
FOOD
BOOK

SUBAH SARAF

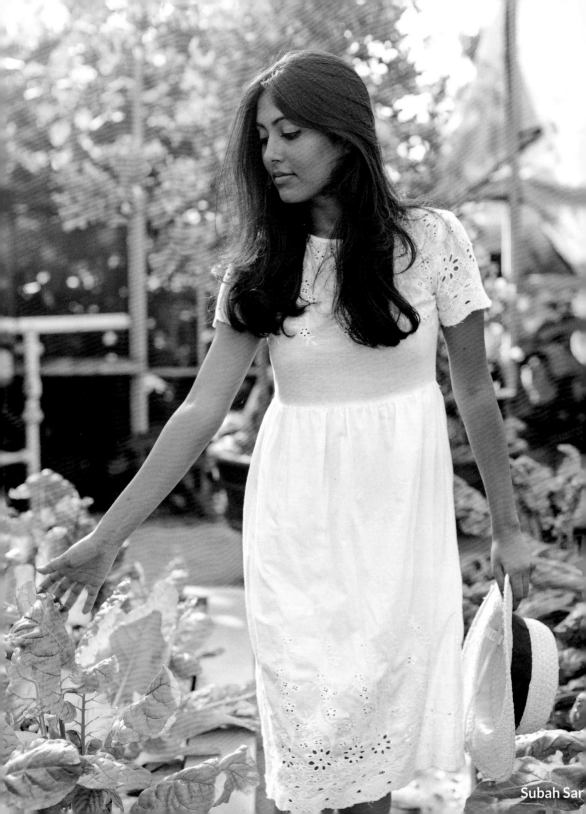
Subah Sar

INDEX

CHAPTER 1

SATVIC FOOD PHILOSOPHY

In this chapter, we will discuss 6 topics -

1. What does Satvic mean?
2. 4 Satvic Food Principles
3. 21 Satvic Food Laws
4. Understanding Digestion
5. Food Combining
6. How you eat is more important than what you eat

What does Satvic mean?

Lord Krishna, in the Bhagavad Gita states that all embodied souls are working under the control of 3 modes, or qualities of material nature -

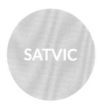 SATVIC
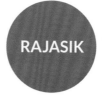 RAJASIK
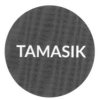 TAMASIK

The thoughts in our head, the activities we perform, the people we meet, the food we eat can all be classified as either Satvic, Rajasik or Tamasik.

Each mode has different characteristics

SATVIC
Mode of Goodness

Purity
Happiness
Compassion
Bliss
Love
Self Control
Satisfaction
Non Violence
Fearlessness
Surrender

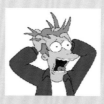

RAJASIK
Mode of Passion

Arrogance
Ego
Restlessness
Anxiety
Anger
Impatience
Fear
Uncontrollable desires
Distress

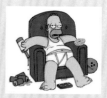

TAMASIK
Mode of Ignorance

Laziness
Tiredness
Depression
Lethargy
Ignorance
Apathy
Inertia
Illusion

One person can have multiple modes

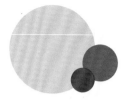
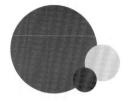
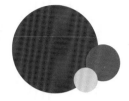

When Satvic dominates, we feel happy, satisfied, & in control of our senses.

When Rajasik dominates, we feel restless, anxious and angry.

When Tamasik dominates, we feel lazy, tired, depressed and lethargic.

Our modern lifestyle, with its high levels of stress and toxins, leads to a life that fluctuates between Rajasik and Tamasik modes. To achieve happiness, we have to transcend from Tamasik and Rajasik to Satvic.

Our food can also be either Satvic, Rajasik or Tamasik

In the 17th chapter of Bhagavad Gita, Lord Krishna explains what Satvic, Rajasik and Tamasik foods are.

Verse 8

āyuḥ-sattva-balārogya-sukha-prīti-vivardhanāḥ
rasyāḥ snigdhāḥ sthirā hṛidyā āhārāḥ sāttvika-priyāḥ

Foods in the mode of goodness increase the duration of life, purify one's existence and give strength, health, happiness and satisfaction. Such foods are juicy, fatty, wholesome, and pleasing to the heart.

Verse 9

katv-amla-lavanaty-usna-tiksna-ruksa-vidahinah
ahara rajasasyesta duhkha-sokamaya-pradah

Foods that are too bitter, too sour, salty, pungent, dry and hot, are liked by people in the modes of passion. Such foods cause pain, distress, and disease.

Verse 10

yata-yamam gata-rasam puti paryusitam ca yat
ucchistam api camedhyam bhojanam tamasa-priyam

Food cooked more than three hours before being eaten, which is tasteless, stale, putrid, decomposed and unclean, is food liked by people in the mode of ignorance.

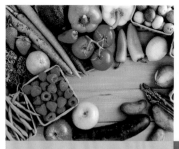 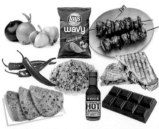 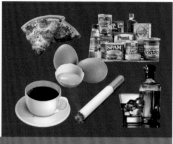

SATVIC FOOD	RAJASIK FOOD	TAMASIK FOOD
Foods that are fresh, wholesome (unprocessed, unrefined), juicy (water-rich), freshly cooked & lightly seasoned are Satvic in nature	Foods that are too bitter, too sour, salty, pungent, dry and hot are Rajasik in Nature	Foods that are stale (eaten after 3 hours of being cooked), rotten (meat and fish) and foul (bad-smelling) are Tamasik in Nature
Satvic Food is living food, with life energy inside it	Rajasik food includes foods with excess flavoring of salt and spices	Tamasik Food is dead. When we eat dead food, the same death is transferred to our body in the form of disease
It is food straight from Nature, with no or minimal human interference		

Examples of Satvic Food	Examples of Rajasik Food	Examples of Tamasik Food
All Fresh Fruits melons, oranges, papaya, apple, pear, berries, grapes, etc.	**Sharp Flavors** excess of salt, red chili, garam masala, asafoetida (*heeng*), vinegars, etc	**Stale Food** everything packaged, bottled, tinned, or canned
All Vegetables bottle-gourd, ridge-gourd, bell peppers, carrots, spinach, coriander, all leafy greens, etc.	**Hot Drinks** very hot water, very hot herbal tea	**Meat, Fish & Eggs** **Stimulants** onion, garlic, tea, coffee, alcohol, cigarettes, betel nut (*supaari*), betel leaf
Whole Fats coconut, soaked nuts & seeds		
Whole Grains whole wheat (with *chokar*), brown rice		

EFFECTS OF SATVIC FOOD

Satvic food is healing food. It is easy to digest, so when we eat it, our body has to spend less time digesting, and can spend more time healing.

By switching to a Satvic diet and lifestyle, we can fully cure any chronic disease, without any medicines.

But the benefits of Satvic food go far beyond the physical body. Gradually, as we keep eating Satvic food, even our thoughts change. It brings mental clarity, calmness and humility. We elevate to a higher consciousness of fearlessness. We become closer to Mother Nature and God.

EFFECTS OF RAJASIK & TAMASIK FOOD

Eating Rajasik and Tamasik food does not only ruin our bodily health, but also our mental health.

If we eat predominantly Rajasik and Tamasik foods, in due course of time, we become a victim of many diseases, such as diabetes, obesity, high blood pressure, PCOD, high cholesterol, joint pains, etc.

On a more subtle level, they have a huge impact on our thoughts. We become arrogant, restless, anxious and impatient. Our concentration levels are decreased and we become dull and lazy. We eat dead foods and hence, our body, emotions and confidence slowly begins to die.

To follow the Satvic diet, we need Satvic recipes and hence we have created this book. Satvic recipes are different from other so-called 'healthy recipes'. They follow strict Satvic food laws and are made especially for healing and achieving the maximum potential of this human body.

4 Satvic Food Principles

According to the Bhagavad Gita, our food should have four qualities, which can be represented by the abbreviation LWPW.

1
LIVING
Our food should come straight from the farm to our kitchen, not go to a factory in between. Nothing processed, tinned, packaged, bottled or canned.

2
WHOLESOME
Our food should be unprocessed & unrefined. It should not have been subtracted of it's natural elements. Whole grains, dates and brown rice are a few examples.

3
PLANT-BASED
Our food should be derived from plants & trees, not from animals. No meat, fish or eggs.

4
WATER-RICH
Our food should be juicy, containing high amount of water, for example - fruits, vegetables, leafy greens. Nuts, seeds, grains are water-poor foods.

Watch the full video on the 4 food principles. Scan the QR code on the left.

1 Our food should be LIVING

Living foods are foods that come straight from Nature, without cooking or processing. Eating living foods means eating foods in their pristine, raw state. To understand this concept better, let's take an example of a wheat plant. If we take a wheat seed, bury it in the soil and water it for a few days, it will grow into a sapling. But if we take wheat noodles and plant them in the ground, will they ever grow into a wheat plant? NO! Because unlike the wheat seed, the noodles do not contain any life energy, or prana. Therefore, they cannot produce more life. They're dead. How can something that is dead bring life to our own body? On the other hand, fruits, vegetables, sprouts, coconut, grains, nuts & seeds (if soaked) are all living foods. When these living foods enter our body, they transfer their life energy inside us, flush out the toxins sitting inside and cure disease.

According to the Bhagavad Gita, chapter 17, verse 10, food should be eaten within 3 hours of being cooked. After 3 hours, it starts to lose the life energy inside it and becomes Tamasik. That explains why in the Yogic Culture, yogis do not eat sabzi, rice or chapati if it has been kept for more than 3 hours. Our forefathers and grandparents also obeyed this law. They used to eat everything fresh - straight from the stove to the plate. However, these days, people store cooked food in the refrigerator for several days, take a little out every day, eat it and store it back. They're eating stale, rotten food. They're inviting cancer into their bodies.

If something is cooked on fire, we must eat it within 3 hours, maximum 5 hours.

But, why only apply this 3-hour-rule to sabzi and chapati? What about all the processed biscuits, chips, candies, snacks and namkeens? Forget 3 hours or even 3 days. Most of them were cooked even 3 years in advance and have been stored in bottles, tins, cans and boxes after being lathered with synthetic chemicals and preservatives. These chemicals might increase the shelf life of these products, but they decrease the shelf life of our own bodies. If you think about it, the processed and packaged stuff we get from factories is not even food. They're products made by a company who wants to make a profit, like any other business. They're dead! They have no life energy left inside.

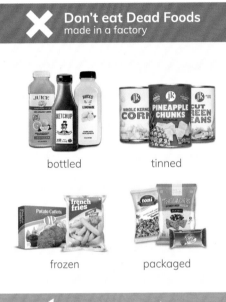

✗ Don't eat Dead Foods
made in a factory

bottled

tinned

frozen

packaged

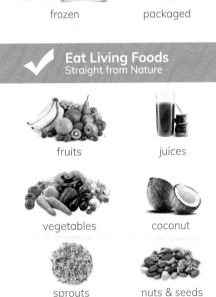

✓ Eat Living Foods
Straight from Nature

fruits

juices

vegetables

coconut

sprouts

nuts & seeds

IT'S NOT UNCOOKED, IT'S SUNCOOKED

At least 70% of our daily diet should consist of raw foods (such as fruits, vegetables, salads, smoothies, juices, sprouts that have not been heated or cooked on fire).

Actually, "sun-cooked" is a more appropriate term than "raw". The term "raw" implies that it is not a finished product, that something is yet to be done. However, a fruit ripening on the tree is certainly not raw food. It may not have been cooked over fire, but it has been cooked by Mother Nature under the sun. It is sun-cooked food. By cooking a fruit or vegetable on the stove, we're actually re-heating it.

Sun is the greatest source of energy on this planet. Sun-cooked, or raw foods carry with them this vibrant sun energy that nourishes all life on Earth. Every whole plant food is a symphony. It is the result of the absorption and accumulation of sun energy.

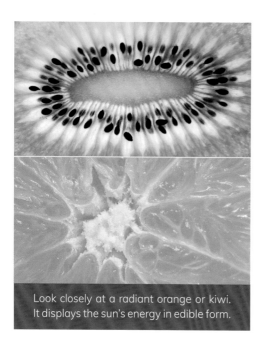

Look closely at a radiant orange or kiwi. It displays the sun's energy in edible form.

When we eat these raw sun foods, their life energy is directly transferred to us, undiminished. This sun energy is used to heal us, rebuild tissues and cells, replace old, damaged or dead cells in our skin and remove cysts, mucus, or stones from our organs. The sun's energy is used to flush out toxins from the body. By eating a diet primarily of raw food, one can overcome any health challenge.

How cooking kills our food?

When we cook our food on fire, the first thing to go is the vital sun-energy. The second thing to go are valuable enzymes in that food. Enzymes are present in all raw foods. Enzymes are what make digestion possible. At 118 degrees Fahrenheit (47.8 degrees Celsius), the enzymes in our food begin to die and the food starts losing it's nutritional value. Food enzyme shortages, sooner or later, result in physical degeneration and disease.

In the Essene Gospel of Peace, Lord Jesus clearly and beautifully explains the impact of dead foods on our body, thoughts and soul.

"Kill neither men, nor beasts, nor yet the food which goes into your mouth. For if you eat living food, the same will quicken you, but if you kill your food, the dead food will kill you also. For life comes only from life, and from death comes always death. For everything which kills your foods, kills your bodies also. And everything which kills your bodies kills your souls also. And your bodies become what your foods are, even as your spirits, likewise, become what your thoughts are. Therefore, eat not anything which fire, or frost, or water has destroyed. For burned, frozen and rotted foods will burn, freeze and rot your body also."

- Jesus, Essene Gospel of Peace

When food is cooked it always becomes less than it was before, never more. Fire is destroyer. it never creates anything. If you light this book on fire, would it become more or less than it was before? Cooking only takes away. It destroys many important nutrients & vitamins in our food.

The assumption behind cooking food is that the original form of Nature, as it exists, must be altered in order that it may be reformed to a new artificial form. The truth is that the original state is always superior. Nothing can compare to the aristocratic taste of a ripe mango, nothing can compare to the taste of fresh watermelons in the summer, nothing even resembles the energy derived from a meal of jack-fruit.

Hence, eat things in nature, the way you find them in nature. Man thinks he is better than nature and that he can improve upon nature. But nature has already perfected it. Anything that we do is only going to lessen the perfection that it's already got.

We understand if you cannot eat a 100% raw diet (although that would be most ideal), but at least strive for 70% of your diet as being fully raw. If you have to cook your food, cook it at the lowest temperatures, for the shortest duration. Steaming is better than boiling. Remove all processed, packaged, tinned, bottled and canned foods from your kitchen. They are the worst, as they have been cooked to death at very high temperatures for long hours. They are dead foods and only transfer death and disease to our own bodies.

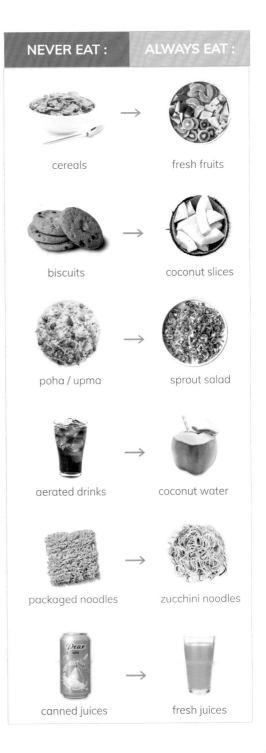

NEVER EAT :   **ALWAYS EAT :**

cereals → fresh fruits

biscuits → coconut slices

poha / upma → sprout salad

aerated drinks → coconut water

packaged noodles → zucchini noodles

canned juices → fresh juices

2 Our food should be WHOLESOME

Mother nature knows best. There's a reason why She hung dates on trees, and not sugar. There's a reason why She gives us coconut, and not coconut oil, potatoes, but not potato chips.

All foods that come directly from plants and trees are wholesome - raw fruits and vegetables for example. They have not been subtracted of anything. Nature has given each food item a specific ratio of protein, fats, nutrients - so that we humans can easily digest and eliminate it.

However, if we fragment it by consuming only a part of it, by stripping away its outer layer, or by squeezing the oil out of it, we are spoiling Nature's original design.

Mother Nature has made each food item a 'whole-package deal'. If she gives us rice, she gives us the mechanism of digesting that rice in the bran that covers it. If we fragment food by throwing out the bran or the roughage, we also throw away the digestive mechanism of that food. White rice, sugar, oils, refined flours, refined wheat - are all highly fragmented foods. They have been highly altered from the way Nature gave them to us. When we eat such unnatural foods, they do not get properly digested in our body, leave undigested residue inside our intestines, leading to disease.

To understand the difference between wholesome and fragmented food clearly, let's take the example of corn. Corn on the cob is obviously whole. Cornmeal is just ground up whole corn - still whole. Dextrose - a sugar that can be made from corn - not whole. And high fructose corn syrup - the king of not being whole.

Eat brown rice instead of white rice. Brown rice is wholesome. When we remove the bran, it becomes white rice. The digestive

mechanism of that rice lies in the outer bran that we conveniently decide to throw out, so the rice can have a longer shelf life.

Eat dates or jaggery instead of sugar. Dates are wholesome. Sugar is fragmented.

Eat whole coconut instead of coconut oil. Eat the whole almond instead of almond oil.

When eating wheat, eat only whole wheat, along with the outer layer, or chokar. Do not sieve it before making your chapatis.

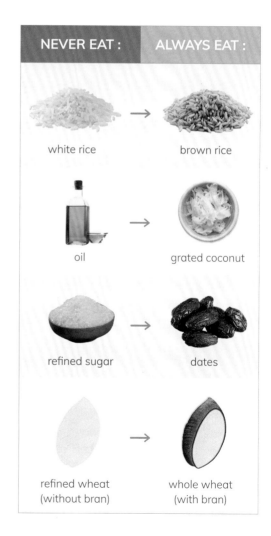

NEVER EAT :	ALWAYS EAT :
white rice	brown rice
oil	grated coconut
refined sugar	dates
refined wheat (without bran)	whole wheat (with bran)

3 Our food should be PLANT-BASED

NATURE HAS NOT DESIGNED THE HUMAN BODY TO EAT MEAT

Nature has constructed every organism either a carnivore (an organism that feeds on other organisms) or a herbivore (an organism that feeds on plants). By looking at our own physical features, we can judge whether we are designed carnivores or herbivores.

	CARNIVORE	HERBIVORE	HUMAN
Teeth	Have sharp, pointed teeth to prey and tear apart meat	Have flat teeth, incapable of tearing apart flesh	Have flat teeth, incapable of tearing apart flesh
Nails	Have sharp, pointed claws to snatch and rip apart flesh	Have flat, dull nails, incapable of tearing flesh	Have flat, dull nails. Have fingers perfectly designed to forge, grab and peel
Intestine Length	Have a very short intestinal tract - only 3-6 times it's body's length. Meat, as a substance is very quick to rot and decompose. A carnivore's digestive tract is short, so the meat exits the body before it becomes toxic	Have a very long intestinal tract - about 12 times it's body's length.	Have a very long intestinal tract. If we eat meat, it does not digest, sits, rots and creates toxicity in the intestines. It grows fungus, mucus and constipation in the intestines.
Stomach Acidity	Have very strong hydrochloric acid in the stomach, to be able to break down meat	Have hydrochloric acid that is almost 20 times weaker than carnivores	Have hydrochloric acid that is almost 20 times weaker than carnivores
Vision	Have eyes that enable them to see even in the dark so they can hunt their prey. Owls, eagles, cats and dogs - they have eyes that shine at night	Do not have night vision, because they are not designed to hunt and prey at night	Do not have night vision, because we are not designed to hunt and prey at night

If Nature had designed meat as our natural food, wouldn't she have given us sharp nails and teeth to tear it apart, shorter intestines, strong hydrochloric acid and night vision eyes? Nature does not make mistakes. Meat is not our natural food.

TOXICITY IN ANIMAL SWEAT

Have you ever had to speak in front of a large audience? Or been in a situation which made you extremely scared or nervous? What was your first reaction to fear? It is to sweat.

Imagine that chicken or pig placed in a row to be slaughtered a moment later. Their fear of death causes a rush of adrenaline through their body, which makes them sweat profusely. Large amounts of toxins are released from the animals cells when it sweats. Regrettably, these toxins remain in the layers between the animal's skin and are served to people in the name of food. If we're eating meat, we're not only eating the flesh of dead animals, but all the toxins that exist in its body. Over the years, these toxins are retained in the blood stream and tissues vitiating the blood, giving rise to inflammation, pain, functional disturbances and degenerative ailments.

OUR STOMACH IS NOT A GRAVEYARD

When a someone dies, we take their body to a cemetery or graveyard to be burnt or buried. But when we consume the dead body of an animal or bird, aren't we making your own stomach a graveyard? Think about it. Our body should be a garden, not a graveyard.

All religions of this world have favored vegetarianism. An innumerable number of people of world wide fame have been vegetarians, such as Plato, Plutarch, Pythogoras, Socrates, Seneca, Zoroaster,

Buddha, Jesus, Hippocrates, Voltaire, Leonardo Da Vinci, Alexander Pope, Tolstoy, Sir Isaac Newton, Thomas Edison, Gandhi, Bernard Shaw and many others. The world's greatest masterpieces, such as the Bhagavad Gita, Zend Avesta of Zoroaster and the Essene Gospel of Peace have advocated a vegetarian diet for man.

'Thou shalt not kill,' for life is given to all by God, and that which God has given, let not man take away. For I tell you truly, from one Mother proceeds all that lives upon the earth. Therefore, he who kills, kills his brother. And from him will the Earthly Mother turn away, and will pluck from him her quickening breasts. And he will be shunned by her angels, and Satan will have his dwelling in his body. And the flesh of slain beasts in his body will become his own tomb. For I tell you truly, he who kills, kills himself, and whoso eats the flesh of slain beasts, eats of the body of death. For in his blood every drop of their blood turns to poison; in his breath their breath to stink; in his flesh their flesh to boils; in his bones their bones to chalk; in his bowels their bowels t o decay; in his eyes their eyes to scales; in his ears their ears to waxy issue. And their death will become his death.

- Jesus, Essene Gospel of Peace

ANIMALS HAVE A REVENGE ON US

What we do always comes back to us. It's called the law of Karma. Even when we kill or eat an animal, the animal has a revenge on us. The revenge is that they slowly begin to kill us, by giving us heart disease, cancer, strokes, etc. It's instant karma.

Dr. William C. Roberts, MD, remarked "When we kill animals to eat them, they end up killing us because their flesh, which contains cholesterol and fat was never intended for human beings, who are natural herbivores." Nowadays, several documentaries are coming up presenting scientific research showing how meat is the leading cause of heart disease, diabetes, obesity and cancer.

Watch the documentaries *Forks Over Knives*, *Food Choices* and *What The Health*.

EFFECTS OF MEAT ON THE MIND

What we eat dramatically affects the way we think. Food has consciousness. We cannot remain positive by ingesting a consciousness of poison, pain and death.

Factory-farmed animals are kept in darkness and squeezed together in inhospitable cages. If we eat the flesh of tortured animals, their energy and consciousness at that time is transferred to us. Not only do we ingest the animal, but also the pain, exhaustion and sorrow of those beings. Our body begins to accumulate that death energy, which manifests within us in the form of anger, violence, depression and illness.

On the other hand, if we take living food and positive, living thoughts, we also become positive and living!

If I don't eat meat, where will I get my protein from?

It is surprising for people to learn that the overconsumption of protein presents a far greater threat to our health than not getting enough. In fact, a major culprit in many diseases is a protein overdose. In order to really be convinced, it is important to know the role of protein in the body.

Protein is a 'building block' for our body. It is needed for the 'growth' of our body. When growth rate is rapid and vast amounts of new cells are being formed, the demand for protein is high. This is during childhood, adolescence, athletes and pregnant women.

When our body reaches adulthood and our height is no longer growing, or if we're living a sedentary lifestyle, our need for protein is minimal, which is easily fulfilled by eating leafy greens, vegetables, fruits, coconut, sprouts, nuts and grains. It's almost impossible to design a protein deficient diet surrounding a variety of whole plant foods.

Any excess than that makes us prone to cancer, formation of cysts, stones and fibroids, unwanted growth hormones and disturbed blood chemistry, amongst many other diseases.

Athletes and children can add soaked nuts and seeds, lentil sprouts, leafy sprouts, coconut, grains, lentils to their diet. Every plant food contains protein. They do not need meat, whatsoever.

Think about it - all the animals that we chose to eat for protein, are vegetarian animals. Where's the logic in that? Do you know that a gorilla can lift something 2,000kg (as heavy as 30 humans), over 10 times it's body weight. Their diet consists of stems, fruits and bamboo shoots. They do not eat meat. Where do they get their protein from? If there was no protein in grass and leaves, how would these animals have been so strong? It makes no sense to go through an animal to get the nutrient that the animal gets, because the animal ate plants.

MILK - to drink or not to drink?

Milk is a complicated subject, so we must deal with it in an orderly way.

According to our scriptures, pure cow milk is not wrong. In fact, producing milk and drinking milk has been sanctioned by God in our scriptures. The problem in not in milk itself, but in what we're getting today in the name of milk today and in our inability to digest it.

There are three problems with animal milk. Let's discuss each one in a logical manner.

1) **Commercial milk is highly adulterated**

The commercial milk that we're getting today is hardly even milk. It is a white-liquid heavily treated with contaminants such as urea, starch, caustic soda, detergents, white paint and refined oil. These contaminants are deliberately added to milk as they provide thickness, preserve milk and increase the volume of milk to make more milk, fast.

We urge you to watch the video linked to the QR code below. The video shows the reality of milk that we drink everyday..

While the immediate effect of drinking such milk range from thyroid disfunctioning, diabetes, gastritis, PCOD, weight gain and high blood pressure, the long-term effects are far more serious.

Can milk adulteration result in cancer?

The World Health Organization (WHO) had recently issued an advisory to the Government of India stating that if adulteration of milk and milk products is not checked immediately, 87 per cent of citizens would be suffering from serious diseases like cancer by the year 2025.

2) **Cows are often mistreated & tortured**

The importance of milk, as described in our scriptures, is fully dependent on cow service. However, today the production of milk has emerged as an industry - one of the most brutal, heartless industries.

For cows to be healthy, they need to be out in fresh air and graze on open fields. However, nowadays, cows are tied to one corner all the time or sometimes even packed in wooden crates. As a result, they fall ill - both physically and emotionally. In hopes of curing them, they are injected with chemical medicines, leading to a downward spiral of disease and depression. If the cows themselves aren't healthy, how can we stay healthy by drinking their milk?

Like any other mother, a cow produces milk for the purpose of feeding its baby calf. However, as soon as the mother gives birth to the calf, they are separated from each other and tied apart. Everyday, the farmer deceives the cow so that she produces milk. He opens the calf and the cow produces milk in its udder for feeding its baby. While the calf is still drinking his mother's milk, the farmer brutally snatches it and ties it away from his mother. Then, the cruel hands of the farmer tie the cows legs and forcefully extract all the remaining milk that was meant for its baby.

For several days, the same process is repeated. When the cow starts understanding that she is being tricked, she becomes restless and starts fighting the farmer so as to say- "Dear farmer, Please let me go. Please don't take away my right to feed my child." The shameless human does not understand. He ties the cow's legs with a rope and continues milking it. After few months, the cow stops producing any milk at all and then, she is injected with a poisonous vaccine that forces her to keep producing milk. This way, the cow is subjected to relentless cycles of exploitation and depression.

Till when will we humans continue to be so brutal towards these innocent, helpless animals? As we discussed earlier, food carries consciousness. Milk that has been obtained by such a devious consciousness, cannot possibly do good to our body.

3) Milk is difficult to digest for those trying to cure a disease or living a sedentary lifestyle

A cow's milk is a very heavy food by nature, designed to create a huge, big boned animal. It contains fast growing steroids and hormones. It is designed to feed an infant calf weighing 90 pounds at the time of birth and 2000 pounds at the age of two. In contrast, a human infant weighs about 6-8 pounds at the time of birth and attains a weight of only 100-200 pounds by the age of 18. Cows milk contains excessive growth promoting hormones.

If we have reached adulthood (we are no longer growing) and if we're not athletes, our body cannot utilize these excessive growth hormones, so it just sits logging our intestines, blood vessels and interrupting blood circulation and absorption, causing many chronic diseases.

If I have access to pure cow milk, can I drink it?

To be qualified to drink milk, there are 8 conditions that must be met -

1. The milk should be obtained from your own farm, or from the farm of a known friend or relative, where you are sure that the cow is loved and cared for.

2. The calf has the first right over that milk. If any milk remains after, only then shall you have it.

3. The cow should be fed good quality grass.

4. The cow should not be injected with any vaccines or chemicals.

5. Even if all 4 laws above prevail, you cannot drink milk if you are trying to heal a disease or living a sedentary lifestyle. You may only drink it if you are an athlete (exercising for more than 3 hours a day) or child whose height is growing.

6. The milk should be preferably raw or at most, boiled lightly only once.

7. The milk should come from cow alone, and no other animal. No buffalo milk. No goat milk.

8. Treat one glassful as milk as a complete meal. Do not combine it with anything.

Milk that complies to all 8 conditions is called **Vedic Milk** and can be consumed only by those doing heavy physical exercise and children. Unfortunately, it is nearly impossible to find such milk in today's day and age. Hence we suggest to abstain from animal milk altogether and switch to another, more digestible replacement.

Is there a replacement for milk?

Indeed, there is. It's coconut milk. Traditionally, coconut has been viewed as India's most sacred fruit. It is the only fruit that has been called 'Shree' Phal in our Vedic scriptures. It's the only fruit that has been attributed with 'Shree' before it.

In India, every auspicious occasion begins

with the breaking of a coconut - marriage, birth, the launch of a house or any other new work. There is a deep significance behind this ritual. Let's understand. Our ancestors were much smarter than us. They knew how nutritious coconut is. However, it was only grown on the coasts of India, but they wanted it to reach every house in India. So they made a ritual stating that no marriage, no birth and no auspicious occasion can begin without the breaking of a coconut. By making it a prerequisite for almost every occasion, it would automatically become a necessity and people found their own ways to transport & spread it throughout the country.

A coconut contains every nutrient that our body needs. Unlike other proteins, coconut is easy to digest. It is superior to all nuts and seeds. It helps underweight people put on healthy weight. There's no cholesterol in raw coconut, unless it is cooked on fire (this is why we never cook coconut directly on stove in Satvic cuisine). Hence, incorporate more coconut in your diet. It is one of Nature's most precious gifts to humanity.

The hard kernel in a mature coconut can be used to make coconut milk. It is very easy and the method of making coconut milk is illustrated on page 49. You can use coconut milk in smoothies, soups, salad dressings.

Make sure to always make coconut milk fresh at home. Do not use the store-bought packaged coconut milk. If you are living in a country where fresh coconuts are not available, you may use homemade almond milk instead (but bear in mind that coconut is more easily digestible than almonds or other nuts).

Almost every animal-based food can be replaced with a more digestible, plant-based food. Let's look at a few replacements.

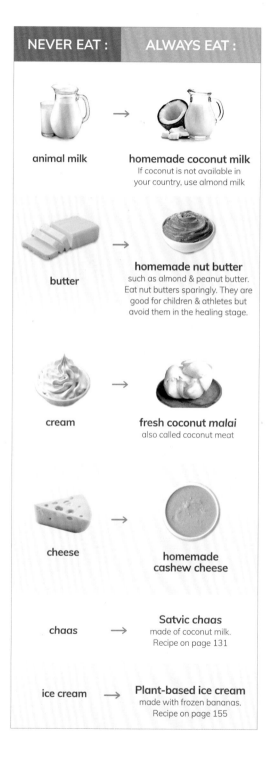

NEVER EAT :   **ALWAYS EAT :**

animal milk → **homemade coconut milk**
If coconut is not available in your country, use almond milk

butter → **homemade nut butter**
such as almond & peanut butter. Eat nut butters sparingly. They are good for children & athletes but avoid them in the healing stage.

cream → **fresh coconut malai**
also called coconut meat

cheese → **homemade cashew cheese**

chaas → **Satvic chaas**
made of coconut milk. Recipe on page 131

ice cream → **Plant-based ice cream**
made with frozen bananas. Recipe on page 155

4. Our food should be **WATER-RICH**

According to the Bhagavad Gita, our food should be juicy, meaning water-rich. Let's understand what water-rich means.

Food can be classified in two categories - water-rich and water-poor.

BEST

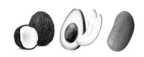

EXTREMELY WATER-RICH
juicy fruits, vegetables, leafy greens

BETTER

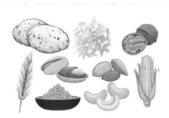

NEUTRAL
fatty fruits, starchy vegetables

GOOD

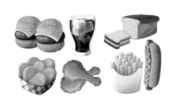

WATER-POOR
grains, legumes, nuts, seeds

WORST

EXTREMELY WATER-POOR
processed food, meat, eggs

Water-rich foods have high-water content. Fruits such as melons, berries, apples, grapes, oranges, tomatoes, cucumbers and vegetables such as bottle gourd, ash gourd, celery and all leafy greens fall in this category. Water-rich foods are light and easy to digest, and are also like laxatives.

Water-poor foods consist of low-water content. Examples include all grains (such as rice, wheat), millets, lentils, beans, and starchy vegetables such as potatoes, yam and all nuts and seeds. These foods are relatively more difficult to digest and can be constipating, unless taken in limited quantities, for those living a sedentary lifestyle.

To identify whether a food is water-rich or water-poor, put it in the juicer. If a lot of juice comes out of it, we know it's water-rich. Can we juice a chapati or rice? No, because there is no juice in it.

The more water a food contains, the easier it is to break down and the quicker it passes through your digestive system. Once the food gets digested, the healing power (*praanshakti*) resumes healing the body and curing disease. On the other hand, water-poor foods are dense. The healing power (*praanshakti*) has to put great effort to break them down. The time that could have been used for healing is diverted to digesting and eliminating these water-poor foods.

In the Bhagavad Gita, chapter 17, verse 8, Lord Krishna describes the qualities of Satvic foods. The first quality of Satvic food, he describes, is to be *rasyāḥ* - meaning juicy in Sanskrit. Such foods increase the duration of life, purify one's existence and give strength, health, happiness and satisfaction, says Lord Krishna.

In the next verse, He also says that foods that are *rūkṣha* (meaning dry (water-poor) in

17

Sanskrit) are Rajasik and are liked by those in the mode of passion. Such foods cause pain, distress, and disease, says Lord Krishna.

Hence we can conclude that water-poor foods eaten in the slightest excess are health destroying and disease promoting, especially for those living a sedentary lifestyle.

Water-poor foods such as beans, lentils, too much grain, may be harmless to bulls, horses, athletes and laborers who work extremely hard, but not to sedentary people or those trying to cure a disease.

What percentage of my diet should be water-rich?

About 70% of our body is water and so, about 70% of our diet should consist of water-rich foods and the remaining 30% can consist of water-poor foods. This is how our daily diet ratio should look like -

30%
Water-Poor
grains, legumes,
nuts, seeds

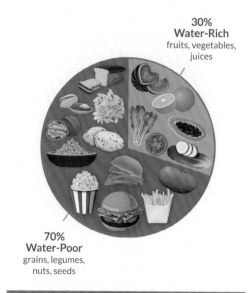

70%
Water-Rich
fruits, vegetables, juices

✔ THE RIGHT RATIO

Funnily enough, most of us eat in the exact opposite ratio -

30%
Water-Rich
fruits, vegetables,
juices

70%
Water-Poor
grains, legumes,
nuts, seeds

✖ THE WRONG RATIO

We have a heavy grain-rich meal 3-4 times a day and as a result, we're drying up!

Let's take the example of a plant. In order to grow optimally, a plant needs both soil and water. Without enough water, the plant dries up, the stems lose their flexibility and branches harden to a point where they can no longer bend and begin to easily break. The human body is made of the same 5 elements as the plant. Just like the plant, when our body doesn't get enough water, it starts losing it's flexibility, our bones degenerate, lose their strength, and here come bone related disorders such as arthritis, rheumatism, cervical, spondylitis, knee pain and back pain.

Just like the plant needs a combination of earth and soil to grow, so does our body.

Mother Nature has generously filled fruits and vegetables with the perfect proportion of soil and water, that can be easily digested by the body.

The meal plans given in this book are designed such that about 70% of your diet is automatically water-rich, starting with juice in the morning, juicy fruits for breakfast, composite chapati (made of 50% vegetable) and satvic sabzi for lunch and a soup / salad for dinner.

In recipes containing rice, wheat or any other grain, the grain has been mixed with double or triple the amount of vegetables (such as in Satvic Daliya, Satvic Khichdi, Coco Quinoa Bowl). Adding a sufficiency of vegetables to grains makes the grain easier to digest.

Lentils and legumes such as kidney beans (rajma), chickpeas (chole) and lentils (daal) have deliberately been avoided in the recipes. It's not that they are wrong foods. It's just that in our modern day sedentary lifestyles, we may not be able to digest them. Our grandparents and forefathers, who spent 8 hours a day in a field doing heavy physical work were able to digest them. But many of us today live a sedentary lifestyle, sitting on an office desk for 8 hours a day, not exercising for more than 1 hour a day. In this situation, it's very difficult to digest kidney beans (rajma), chickpeas (chole) and too much lentil (daal).

FREQUENTLY ASKED QUESTIONS

How much water should I drink in a day?

The answer is simple. Drink water only when you feel thirsty. Nowadays, people are advised to drink 8-10 glasses of water everyday, or 2 glasses immediately after waking up. This is not right because excessive drinking of water puts undue pressure on the kidneys. Instead of digesting the previously eaten meal, the body's energy redirects itself to process all that unnecessary water. When you start following the Satvic food system, you will be eating lots of fruits and salads (with minimal spices and salt) so your need for plain water will reduce substantially, yet there will still be more water going inside you.

I drink coffee, soda and beer. They contain water, don't they?

No. These kinds of drinks act as diuretics—they cause increased passing of urine and actually cause us to lose water and become dangerously dehydrated.

21 Satvic Food Laws

Here are 21 food laws you must follow. All recipes given in this book have been carefully created to adhere to these laws. Please follow every single law religiously to receive the true benefit of the Satvic lifestyle.

	✗	✓
Law 1	**No Animal Based Foods** such as meat, fish, eggs, animal milk*, cheese, butter, ghee, paneer	**Eat Plant Based Foods** such as fresh homemade coconut milk, almond milk
Law 2	**No Dead Foods** Don't eat anything that comes packaged, bottled, tinned or canned from a factory, such as chips, namkeens, snacks, vinegar, soya sauce, ready-made sauces or dressings	**Eat Fresh Foods** Eat foods that come straight from the farm to the kitchen, such as fresh fruits, vegetables, grains, nuts and seeds.
Law 3	**No Sugar** such as white sugar, brown sugar, sugar-syrups, *khaand*, maple syrup, agave	**Use Natural Sweeteners** such as fresh fruits, dates, jaggery, figs, raisins
Law 4	**No White Rice**	**Eat Brown Rice**
Law 5	**No oils** Olive oil, mustard oil, coconut oil, palm oil, refined oil, flaxseed oil, etc.	**Use Whole Fats** Grated fresh coconut, soaked nuts and seeds
Law 6	**No Refined Flours** such as white flour, *maida*, semolina (*sooji*), etc	**Use Whole Flours** whole wheat flour (with *chokar*)
Law 7	**No Red Chili or Red Chili Powder**	**Use Fresh Green Chili or Black Pepper** in limited amounts

*allowed only in few exceptional cases

Law 8	**No Strong Spices** such as garam masala, asafoetida (*heeng*), black salt (*kala namak*), too much ginger, too much salt	**Use Fresh Herbs** such as tulsi, curry leaves, coriander, basil, lemongrass, oregano, rosemary, thyme, bay leaf. Some mild spices such as cardamom, cinnamon and cumin seeds can be used in moderation
Law 9	**No Iodised Salt**	**Use Rock Salt (*Sendha Namak*)** in limited amounts
Law 10	**No Excessive Cooking** Nothing should be cooked too much or for too long, so as to destroy the natural composition of that food. Frying and over-cooking is strictly prohibited.	**Minimal Cooking** Eat most of your food raw. If needed, cook only minimally, for the shortest duration possible • Vegetables & grains can be cooked • Fruits should not be cooked (no cooking tomato, coconut or coconut milk) • Sprouts should not be cooked • Steaming is better than boiling. It preserves more nutrition
Law 11	**No Metal Pots & Pans** for cooking	**Use only Clay Pots & Pans** for cooking
Law 12	**Don't Eat Much Grain** Wheat, rice, lentils, quinoa, millets all come under the umbrella of grains. A satvic dish should not have too many grains, as they are difficult to digest.	**Eat Less Grain, More Vegetables** Maintain a 70-30 ratio between vegetables & grains. If your dish has 30% grains, combine it with at least 70% vegetables. If eating one composite chapati (pg 73), eat with 2 bowls of Satvic sabzi. If eating 2 composite chapatis, eat with 4 bowls of Satvic sabzi. If eating 1 bowl of brown rice, eat with 3 bowls of vegetables.

Law 13

Do Not Mix Multiple Grains in the Same Dish

It is difficult enough for our body to digest one type of grain at a time. If we mix two or more grains together, it becomes even more difficult. So -

- No rice with chapati
- No daal with rice
- No daal with chapati
- No multi-grain flour

Eat Only One Type of Grain at a Time

If eating grains, eat with a sufficiency of vegetables, without mixing with another grain.

- Brown Rice with sabzi
- Composite chapati with sabzi
- Quinoa with vegetables

Law 14

No Unseasonal or Exotic Foods

Do not use ingredients that are out of season or are not locally grown in your country, as they tend to contain more chemicals to extend their shelf life.

Ingredients such as blueberries, kale, swiss chard, hazelnuts, macadamia nuts are not local to India, so don't bother using them.

Eat Foods that are Seasonal & Local

Eat foods that are local to your country and are in season. Seasonal fruits and vegetables tend to be cheaper in price.

Law 15

Do Not Use Unsoaked Nuts

Don't use or eat any nuts before soaking them in water.

Use Soaked Nuts

Always soak nuts for 6-8 hours before using. Before being soaked, nuts are in their dormant state Adding water brings them to life and makes them digestible.

Law 16

Do Not Eat Too Many Nuts & Seeds

Similar to grains, nuts & seeds and are difficult to digest and therefore, should be only consumed sparingly. If using nuts in a salad dressing, use only the minimum amount required, for the sake of texture.

Consume Nuts & Seeds Sparingly

If you are trying to cure a disease, it is best to avoid them altogether. Once you are cured, you may have them sparingly (about 5-7 a day). Bear in mind, we have already added them to our salads and salad dressing recipes. If you are eating those, no need to consume nuts/seeds separately.

Law 17

Coconut Milk is superior to almond milk, cashew milk & other nut milks, because coconut is easier to digest than other nuts. So, always prefer fresh homemade coconut milk over other nut milks.

Law 18

No Soy Milk, No Tofu
Soya is very difficult to digest. It is an inferior quality of grain.

Law 19

Coconut & Tomato Should Not Be Cooked Directly on Flame

If adding fresh coconut, coconut milk or tomato in a recipe, add it towards the end, AFTER switching off the stove. You can let the coconut and tomato warm from the steam inside the pot, but never cook them directly on flame.

This also means that after adding coconut, coconut milk or tomato to a dish, it should not be re-heated.

Law 20

In cooked recipes, **add salt and lemon towards the end**, not beginning. Salt and lemon should not be cooked on flame.

Law 21

Do not add grains (such as wheat, rice, millet, lentil) to a salad or soup. Salads and soups should be grain-free, unless they are being eaten as a grain meal.

Understanding Digestion

Essential to the maintenance of physical, mental and emotional health is the timely elimination of toxins that either enter the body or are created by it. Everything in nature follows a specific order & timing. For example, the moon and the sun have regular cycles twelve months of the year; the four seasons are constant & prompt; seeds must sprout before they become plants; fruit trees must blossom before they bear the immature and then the ripened fruit. Our body is a part of nature. Just like nature, our bodies too follow a specific order & timing. The correctness of this order & timing determines our health.

YOU, YOUR WASHING MACHINE & CYCLES

Imagine you are a washing machine. And this washing machine has three mini-cycles, within each complete cycle:

1. Fill and wash
2. Rinse
3. Spin

Similarly, the following mini-cycles are a part of your body's functioning:

1. Digestion
2. Assimilation
3. Elimination

Let's take a look at what happens in a washing machine in regards to these mini-cycles:

- If you allow the washing machine to complete three mini-cycles, your clothes will be bright, clean and fresh.

- If you stop the washing machine just

  before the spin, the clothes remain soaking wet. When they dry, they remain somewhat dirty from the retained water.

- If you stop the washing machine after

  it finishes the wash cycle, the clothes remain full of detergent and dirt.

Therefore:

- If you skip one or more of the mini-cycles, your clothes will be less clean than you expect. You can blame this deficiency on your washing machine, but of course you are responsible.

What does this have to do with the cycles of digestion, absorption and elimination? Every time you eat a meal, a significant portion of your body's energy shifts from whatever it was doing, to digesting the food that has entered your stomach. When your body finishes digesting the food, it shifts its energy to absorption. Having completed that, the body's energy proceeds to eliminate waste. All of this works wonderfully unless you eat before the body has finished absorbing or eliminating your most recent meal. When you eat before the most recent meal has been "processed" completely, the body shifts its energy to address the new food. The residue of the most recent meal is then left at the mercy of bacteria, yeast, mold, etc., and the result is the unnecessary production of waste, or, toxins in the body.

Most of us constantly consume before it is time to nourish. Following are the most frequent responses to the question, "When do you decide to eat?"

- "The clock indicates that it is time to eat."
- "I'm bored and have nothing else to do."
- "Every time I see or smell food."

None of these rationalizations justify the eating of excessive food. One should eat when he/she feels true hunger, after the last meal has been digested, absorbed and eliminated.

When you eat a new meal while your body is still assimilating or eliminating the previous meal, you stress and compromise your body unduly, because it is aware that it has not finished its task from the last meal yet has another job requiring immediate commencement. So, the body deals with both meals incompletely, thus generating both excess stress and unnecessary waste.

Most people (in so-called "advanced societies") have pounds of undigested waste stored in their bodies. If you would simply stop eating, the body would be able to finish the work that it began.

Fortunately, the body is very efficient and resilient. It has a powerful will to live. It has an incredible reserve of vital force to maintain relatively good health even when you impede it from fulfilling its natural functions. It usually takes years of abuse to render the human body incapable of rectifying the unhealthy habits that have been imposed upon it.

USING THIS MODEL IN YOUR LIFE

You can apply the cited model to the emotional, mental and spiritual challenges you face. Many gifted people have recognized that healing occurs in a void (the absence of everything). You must leave enough space between events to prevent the second event from running into, over, around or through the first event. Finish processing the first before you commence the next – don't leave unfinished responsibilities to commence new ones. This is a critical lesson that we must learn from life, and when we heed it, we reap bountiful rewards.

LESSONS TO BE LEARNED

What can you do to help your body follow the right eating pattern?

Follow Intermittent Fasting (also called 16 hour fasting) when you eat within a span of 8 hours, and fast for 16 hours every night. This would give your digestive system not only adequate time to finish the cycles, but also adequate time to heal thereafter.

For example, if you eat your dinner at 8pm, eat no solid food till 12 noon the next day. At 12 noon, have your first solid meal of food. If you eat dinner at 6pm, eat no solid food till 10 am the next morning. Water and juices (such as coconut water, ash gourd juice) is allowed in your fasting cycle.

When you do intermittent fasting, your body will digest & absorb food within 5-6 hours (depending on the quality of your food). Once digestion is complete, what does it start doing? It starts healing. In the healing state, it rebuilds old tissue, burns fat cells, fades away old scars and cures your disease.

We have made a video explaining the concept of 16 hour fasting in detail. To watch it, scan the QR code below.

Food Combining

Pairing food in the right way can make all the difference to our digestion. Even fresh, wholesome food, if paired incorrectly, can overwhelm the digestive system and cause indigestion, fermentation, gas, bloating, and the creation of toxins. This is why proper food combining is so important.

Foods are natural chemicals. For the sake of understanding, imagine your body similar to a test tube in a laboratory. As in other chemical experiments, reactions ranging from sedative to explosive can be created in our bodies, depending upon the combination of elements. The more ingredients there are in a meal, the greater the chance for a digestive explosion.

ANALOGY

Imagine a highway. Three categories of vehicles can enter this highway –

1. Scooters
2. Cars
3. Trucks

Scooters are fast. They move quickly through the highway. Trucks are heavier and move very slowly. Cars fall somewhere in between - neither too slow, nor too fast.

This highway can be compared to our digestive tract. Scooters represent fruits – light and quick. Cars represent vegetables. Trucks represent grains - heavy and slow.

On an average, fruits take about of 3 hours to digest and eliminate. Vegetables take a little longer - about 6 hours. Grains (such as wheat, rice, lentils, millets) take about 18 hours to digest, absorb and eliminate from our body. This explains why we often feel lazy and sleepy after eating too many grains, because all our energy goes into digesting it and little remains to keep us awake.

Of course these timings are just estimates to give us an idea. They vary from person to person, age to age, but the point is - the more water in a food substance, the faster it passes through our digestive system. Grains, nuts, seeds, dried fruits are water-poor foods and hence take longer to digest. Fresh fruits, vegetables and juices are water-rich foods and digest and eliminate quickly. For optimum health, at least 70% of our diet should be composed of water-rich foods.

Note

- Legumes, nuts and seeds also take about 18 hours to digest.
- Neutral vegetables (such as lettuce, celery, spinach, coriander, cucumber) are quicker to digest than starchy vegetables (such as potato, peas, pumpkin, cauliflower).

Six Laws of Food Combining

Now that we have learnt about the digestibility levels of different foods, let's understand the laws of food combining.

1 Restrict to eating grain only once a day

As stated before, grains (wheat, rice, lentils, legumes, millets, quinoa) take an average of 18 hours to digest, assimilate and eliminate from the body. If we eat grains twice, or thrice a day – a practice commonly observed amongst Indians– it means that even before our previous grain meal was digested, we give our body more to digest. Then, instead of finishing the digestion of the previous meal, our body shifts its energy to address the new food that has just entered the stomach. The residue of the previous meal is then left at the mercy of bacteria, yeast, mold, etc., and results in the accumulation of undigested food, or waste in the body.

DIFFICULT TO DIGEST COMBINATIONS

- Lentil pancakes (cheela) for breakfast, rice for lunch, sabzi-roti for dinner
- Poha (puffed rice) for breakfast, sabzi-roti for lunch, daal (lentils) for dinner

EASY TO DIGEST COMBINATIONS

- Fruits for breakfast, Satvic sabzi-roti for lunch, salad for dinner
- Fruits for breakfast, salad for lunch, Satvic cheela for dinner
- Salad for breakfast, brown Rice and vegetables for lunch, fruits for dinner

Note Children, athletes, and people engaged in rigorous physical work can afford to eat grains more than once a day, because their digestive powers are stronger than others.

2 Eat only one grain at a time

In our modern day, sedentary (always-sitting) lifestyles, it is difficult enough for the body to digest one grain at a time. If we give it two grains at once, it becomes even more difficult, and many a times, even impossible. So, eat only one grain at a time. If eating chapati, eat only chapati, with a sufficiency of vegetables. Don't eat rice and chapati in the same meal. If eating brown rice, eat only brown rice, mixed with a sufficiency of vegetables.

DIFFICULT TO DIGEST COMBINATIONS

- Rice with chapati (wheat)
- Rajma (kidney beans) with rice
- Daal (lentils) with rice
- Chana (chickpeas) with rice

EASY TO DIGEST COMBINATIONS

- Brown Rice with Vegetables
- Chapati with Vegetables
- Sprouted daal (lentils) with salad

3 When eating grains, mix them with 3 times the vegetables

When making chapati, instead of using 100% wheat flour, use 50% wheat flour and 50% vegetable (such as spinach, carrot, cucumber, beetroot, fenugreek, etc). The method of making composite chapati has been clearly explained later in this book. If eating one chapati, eat 2 bowls of vegetable (sabzi). If eating 2 chapatis, eat 4 bowls of vegetable (sabzi). Adding a sufficiency of vegetables to grains makes the grains easy to digest.

DIFFICULT TO DIGEST COMBINATIONS

- 3 chapatis with 1 bowl of vegetable

EASY TO DIGEST COMBINATIONS

- 1 composite chapati with 2 bowls of vegetable
- 1 bowl of brown rice with 3 bowls of vegetables
- 1 bowl of quinoa with 3 bowls of vegetables

4 Do not eat fruits & cooked food in the same meal

Fruits require different types of enzymes and acid secretions to be released by the stomach than cooked vegetables and grains. Fruits digest best by themselves or with "neutral" green vegetables. The "neutral" vegetables (such as lettuce, cucumber, coriander, celery, and kale) are so called because their starch and fat content is low and, thus, their digestion will not interfere with the digestion of fruit.

DIFFICULT TO DIGEST COMBINATIONS

- Fruits & cooked vegetables in the same meal
- Fruits & grains in the same meal

EASY TO DIGEST COMBINATIONS

- Fruits alone
- Fruits with neutral green vegetables

5 Don't mix sweet fruits with citric fruits

Sweet fruits (mangoes, bananas, *chikoo*, persimmons, etc.) should not be combined with citric fruits (oranges, mandarin, pineapple, lemons), since they require different digestive juices to be released by the stomach. It is best to eat similar kinds of fruits together.

Note   Bulkier fruits like banana, coconut and avocado require more digestion time.

EASY TO DIGEST COMBINATIONS

- Any one single fruit
- Only Melons (Watermelons, Muskmelons, Honeydew Melons)
- Apple, Pear and Peach
- Berries (most)
- Oranges and Mandarin

6 Don't drink while you eat

If you're eating solid foods, stick to solids; conversely, if you're drinking liquids, stick to liquids. Drinking anything while eating dilutes the digestive juices, and causes indigestion. Let us explain how. As soon as we put food in our mouth, a digestive fire lights up inside the stomach to break it down. If we gulp down a glass of water immediately after eating, we extinguish that fire, which was necessary to digest the food. The undigested food rots and causes disease in the body. It is best to drink water at least 1 hour before or 2 hours after our solid meal. Once we start eating Satvic food, which is rich in water and low in spices & salt, we do not feel the need to drink water with or after meals. If drinking water becomes necessary while or after eating food, sip 2 sips of water & let it stay in the mouth for a while before swallowing it. You will not feel thirsty after that.

SURPRISING FACTS

- There are 28 ingredients in an "average" cake mix bought from a store.
- The conventional "festive-meal" in India includes more than 100 ingredients in various combinations.

How you eat is more important than what you eat

Recipes aren't all we need. Here are some simple life skills that can help us live and eat in a more pleasant way.

1 Eat 70% raw, 30% cooked

If you take an apple & plant it in the ground, you're going to get an apple tree. But if you cook that apple, and plant it in the ground, you won't get anything. Once you cook your food, it's dead. Nature has designed our body to take whole foods and eat them in their raw, uncooked form. Every single creature on earth except humans, and the poor animals we've captured, eat a 100% raw diet. Some Health institutes around the world are putting people on a 100% raw diet and reversing even third stage diseases (cancer, tumors, TB, etc). There is yet another advantage of eating raw food. We consume much less of the same food when it is not cooked. Take cauliflower. The average person could not even eat half of a raw cauliflower. But if it were cooked,the same person could easily eat the entire vegetable. By eating uncooked food, we save food, and time in preparing it. It is difficult to follow a completely raw lifestyle but make sure at least 70% of your diet is raw. This is possible if you eat not more than one cooked meal a day, exactly how we've suggested in your meal plan (Pg 55). When preparing cooked food, always cook on a low flame for as little time as possible and try eating within 3 hours of preparing. Never store cooked food in the refrigerator to consume the next day.

> *"Therefore, eat not anything which fire, or frost, or water has destroyed. For burned, frozen and rotted foods will burn, freeze and rot your body also."*
>
> **~ Jesus, Essene Gospel of Peace**

2 Always rest after a grain meal

Picture in your mind a portable mobile phone power bank. If you plug in one phone, all power in the bank will go towards charging that one phone. It will be charged quickly & efficiently. If you plug in 3 phones simultaneously, the energy will get distributed amongst the 3 phones and each phone will be charged less efficiently. Your body works in a similar manner. You receive a limited reserve of power when you wake up every morning. Each action you perform (breathing, talking, walking) takes up an amount of energy from this daily reserve. The greatest expenditure of energy occurs in the work of food digestion. It takes upto 70% of your body's energy. If you perform another taxing task while your food is being digested, your body will not receive enough energy to digest food. Hence, the meal will be left undigested and in due course, set up serious diseases. Life cannot simultaneously carry out adequately more than one great activity - whether it's a physical activity or a mental one. We recommend taking a 30 minute nap, or rest after your grain meal. You need not rest after eating a light meal, such as fruits or smoothies, as they require little energy to digest. If your job doesn't allow time to rest after lunch, eat a lighter lunch and your grain meal at dinner.

> *"Work and digestion must be kept apart, so there may be no competition between them."*
>
> **~ Acharya K. Lakshmana Sarma, Father of Nature Cure in India**

3 Never overeat

Overeating is a curse. Immoderation in matters of diet–either eating too much in every meal or eating too often– leads to deterioration of health and reduces the span of life. Always leave the table a little hungry. Many cultures have rules that tell you to stop eating before you are full. In Japan, they say "eat until you are four fifths full." Islamic culture has similar rule. Germans say "tie off the sack before it's full." If you fill a blender till the top, would it be able to blend? No, because it needs some empty space to twist and turn the ingredients inside. Similarly, if you fill your stomach till the top, will it be able to break down and digest your food? No, because it needs empty space to release and mix digestive juices with the food, and allow for the expansion and contraction of the stomach. Even wholesome food, if eaten in excess, becomes toxic filth. That the minimum food, the food that is needed for replacement of wasted body substance, gives the best result in health, is the conclusion arrived at by all the pioneers and their successors. On the other hand, every excess over this minimum lowers the health-level and provokes disease.

"And when you eat, never eat unto fulness"… "give heed to how much you have eaten when your body is sated, and always eat less by a third"

~ Jesus, Essene Gospel of Peace

4 Eat only when you're hungry

Eating when not really hungry is just adding a load to the body it doesn't need. One should make sure that the following events have been completed before eating a meal - (1) Emptying of the stomach indicated by the elimination of the wastes, (2) Adequate time for rest and recuperation for the organs after elimination, (3) The feeling of bodily lightness and presence of sufficient digestive power to digest the new meal. Those that disregard these rules and eat while stools are stagnant in the bowels, are conservancy carts, carrying the foul refuse of three of four days eating or perhaps a great deal more. They are welcoming serious diseases by doing so. Unless the stomach – not the mind – answers that it's ready for more food, do not eat. Most people eat for the two t's, that is, for the tongue and for the time. Instead, we should eat for the third t: the tummy. Convince your mind that it is ok to skip meals. These mini-fasts can be very beneficial to your health. Airplane travels and other nutritional wastelands are great places to eat less. Of course we advise this within reason. If you are underweight, consistent nutrition is important. Please use good judgment.

"The body will never need medicine if food is never taken without making sure that the stomach has digested what was given to it before."

~ Thiruvalluvar, Great Indian Saint

5 Eat a light breakfast

If breakfast cannot be renounced altogether, it should be a light meal, fruit, or salad, for example. This line of reasoning surprises many Americans, because they are taught from a young age that it's important to begin the day with a hearty breakfast–the "breakfast of champions" approach. But from the yogic perspective, when we first wake up, our digestive fire is not very strong; it's still partly asleep, so our morning meal should be light. Before the white men came, the rule was, at least for the Brahamanas, to go without food till noon, meanwhile doing all the day's work. Professors taught, and pupils learnt their lessons on an empty stomach, and there was a high level of scholarship. In one of our Vedic books there is a passage that says, "Take water and do thy work". Morning eating is also condemned in the Old Testament of the Bible.

Lunch, however, can be a heavier meal, since we have plenty of energy to digest by the time it's noon. Supper, like breakfast, should be light, and we should finish the evening meal at least two hours before going to sleep.

"Sleep is not a hunger inducing process."
~ Dr. Dewey

6 Always eat in a relaxed state

We are not machines. We are a confluence of the body, mind and soul. We should make sure to eat when our body and mind are relaxed; it's best not to eat when we're upset, angry, agitated or in a hurry. Food eaten in such conditions will not be digested, because more of our vital energy will get used to handle the mental stress, and less will remain to carry out the bodily functions, namely digestion. What we don't digest often turns into bacterial fermentation, toxic filth or fat. Make sure you are seated and take the time to enjoy your meal in a relaxed state with a good intention.

Our Indian culture also certifies this principle. If someone dies in a family, cooking is prohibited until the dead body is cremated because in the case of tension and stress, the family member's food does not get digested.

"for all that you eat in sorrow, or in anger, or without desire, becomes a poison in your body." ~ Jesus, Essene Gospel of Peace

7 Don't mix too much together

When you eat just one type of fruit, vegetable or grain, your body digests the food more easily and assimilates it better. When eating fruit, try having similar types of fruits together – for example watermelons with muskmelons, apples with pears, strawberries with raspberries, oranges with other citric fruits. When eating grains, don't mix two different grains in the same meal. For example – don't mix rice with wheat. Instead, eat rice with vegetables, or wheat with vegetables. Don't combine raw and cooked foods at the same meal, as they are broken down differently. Additionally, if you're eating solid foods, stick to solids; conversely, if you're drinking liquids, have only liquids. Your stomach will be grateful to you, because it will have just one thing to do; digestion will be much quicker and easier. Why? Because each food requires a different amount of time to digest and utilizes different digestive juices from the stomach.

"Be content with two or three sorts of foods, which you will find always upon the table of our Earthly Mother."… "For I tell you truly, if you mix together all sorts of food in your body, then the peace of your body will cease, and endless war will rage in you."

~ Jesus, Essene Gospel of Peace

8 Eat neither too cold, nor too hot

The temperature of the food we eat should match the temperature of our own body. Do not eat food that is too hot or too cold; it affects the digestive system negatively. If a food or drink is too hot or too cold, keep it on your tongue for 10-12 seconds before swallowing it. The mouth neutralizes the temperature of anything that you leave inside for that duration. All recipes in this book should be served at room temperature.

"Shun all that is too hot and too cold. For it is the will of your Earthly Mother that neither heat nor cold should harm your body."

~ Jesus, Essene Gospel of Peace

9 Eat Seasonal, Regional and Reasonable

Mother Nature is much smarter than us. There's a very specific reason as to why She gives us certain foods in summer, and not in winter, and vice-versa. When we eat unseasonal fruits and vegetables, we tamper with her plan and this is what leads to all diseases in the modern day. Also, unseasonal fruits are highly contaminated because they require enormous amounts of chemicals and pesticides to be grown out of their season. Secondly, eat regional – food growing in your own country or area. The universe has a place for everything and everything is best suited for where the universe puts it. Imported produce suffers from lengthy transport time and as a result, contains more preservatives to increase it's shelf life. When something is produced in an area at the time when it is in season there, the cost of the food will automatically go down, hence making it reasonable.

"Eat not unclean foods brought from far countries, but eat always that which your trees bear. For your God knows well what is needful for you, and where and when."

~ Jesus, Essene Gospel of Peace

10 Chew, chew & chew

The rule is that one should chew each mouthful so well that food is broken into small particles and becomes well mixed with the saliva of the mouth. Remember, the flow of saliva in the mouth depends on how much you chew your food. That is, the more thorough the chewing, the more the saliva produced, the easier it will be to digest food. The reverse is equally true. In other words, food which is thoroughly chewed is well digested by the organs lower down. In eating by this rule, less is eaten in more time; and so one cannot overeat.

"Nature will castigate those who do not masticate."

~ Horace Fletcher, The Great Masticator

CHAPTER 2

SETTING UP A SATVIC KITCHEN

In this chapter, we will discuss 6 topics -

1. Ingredients needed for a perfect Satvic kitchen
2. 8 essential tools for a perfect Satvic kitchen
3. How to use the tools?
4. All about vegetable sprouts
5. All about nut milks
6. Do's and dont's of recipe making

Ingredients Needed
for a perfect Satvic Kitchen

In order to make the Satvic recipes with ease, it's important to have a well-stocked Satvic Kitchen. Below we have given a list of all ingredients used in this book. We recommend that you buy fruits, vegetables and fresh herbs as and when you make the recipes, but buy all the dry ingredients in advance, in one grocery trip. You will be able to find most ingredients at your common grocery store, or online, on Amazon.

FRESH INGREDIENTS
Buy as & when you make recipes

1. FRUITS   Make sure whatever you buy is seasonal & regional. Do not buy frozen fruits.

- Lemon
- Melons
- Papaya
- Coconut
- Apple

- Pear
- Orange
- Mango
- Banana
- Pomegranate

- Peach
- Berries
- Grapes
- Sapota (*chikoo*)
- Pineapple

2. VEGETABLES   Avoid precut, prepackaged vegetables that have been sitting in plastic bags and containers for who knows how long.

- Ash Gourd
- Bottle Gourd
- Ridge Gourd
- Spinach
- Lettuce
- Rocket leaves
- Cucumbers

- Celery
- Parsley
- Zucchini
- Tomatoes
- Bell Peppers
- Beetroot
- Carrots

- Pumpkin
- Cabbage
- Peas
- Broccoli
- Green Beans
- Cauliflower
- Potatoes

3. HERBS   Growing your own herbs is easy and economical. If you have more than you can use, just dry them and store in jars for future use.

- Coriander
- Mint
- Bay Leaf

- Curry Leaves
- Thyme
- Oregano

- Rosemary
- Lemongrass
- Basil

DRY INGREDIENTS
Buy in advance

1. NUTS AND SEEDS Buy what you'll use within a month and store them in the refrigerator during the summer months. Always soak your nuts and seeds in water before using them.

- Almonds
- Walnuts
- Cashews
- Pistachios

- Peanuts
- Pumpkin Seeds
- Sunflower Seeds
- Poppy Seeds

- Chia Seeds
- Flax Seeds
- Sesame Seeds

2. SEEDS FOR SPROUTING We recommend eating sprouts of vegetable seeds, instead of lentils, because vegetable sprouts are easier to digest. Seeds for sprouting are same as those used to grow the vegetable. You can find them online.

- Alfalfa
- Clover

- Fenugreek
- Radish

3. GRAINS AND LEGUMES

- Whole Wheat Flour
- Brown Rice

- Quinoa
- Moong Daal

- Millets

4. SPICES AND CONDIMENTS

- Rock salt (*sendha namak*)
- Green chillies
- Fresh ginger
- Cinnamon
- Green cardamom buds

- Fennel seeds
- Cumin
- Black pepper
- Saffron strands
- Cacao Powder

- Cacao Nibs
- Galangal
- Vanilla Powder

5. DRY HERBS You can easily find them at grocery stores.

- Dried Basil
- Dried Oregano

- Dried Rosemary
- Dried Thyme

6. SWEETENERS Remove all processed sugars from your kitchen & replace with natural ones.

- Dates
- Raisins

- Chemical Free Jaggery

8 Essential Tools
for a perfect Satvic Kitchen

It is truly a joy to have good kitchen equipment. I recommend that you start with the equipment that you already have, and then every few weeks, purchase one tool that you need.

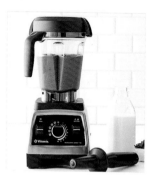

1. Blender

A blender is needed for everything - soups, dressings, nut milks. The recipes in this book will work just fine with an average household blender. But, I recommend you to invest in a high-speed blender. It can make the silkiest sauces, smoothies, soups and creams in very little time. The two most popular high-speed blenders in the market are the Vita-Mix and the Blendtec. High-speed blenders are more expensive, but a great investment if you have any sort of culinary passion.

2. Juicer

You will need to drink lots of juices in your journey of following a Satvic diet. There are two main types of juicers:

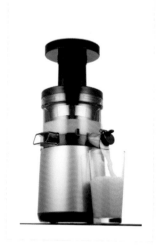

1. Centrifugal Juicers
    These typically utilize a fast-spinning metal blade that separates the juice from flesh via centrifugal force. The problem with centrifugal juicers is that the fast-spinning metal blade generates heat, which destroys the enzymes in the fruits and vegetables you're juicing, leading to a less nutritious juice.

2. Slow Juicers (also known as Cold press Juicers)
    Slow Juicers extract juice by first crushing and then pressing fruit and vegetables for the highest juice yield. Because they don't produce as much heat, they keep more of the nutrients intact, leading to a high quality juice.

If you want to pack the most nutrients in your body as possible, buy a slow press juicer. There is a variety of slow juicers available in the market.

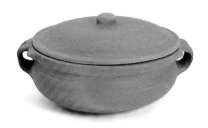

3. Clay Pot

Cooking vegetables, sabzis or rice in a clay pot is much better than cooking in any kind of a metal pot. Clay is porous in nature, it allows moisture and heat to circulate through your food, and thus, retain its nutrition. Food cooked in a clay pot even tastes better. Our ancestors all used clay pots to cook their food. Clay pots are inexpensive and are easily available in local Indian markets, or online. If clay pots are not available, use stainless steel vessels (without nickel plating). Do not use aluminum or non-stick cookware.

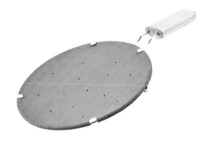

4. Clay Tawa

A clay tawa is essential for those who want to cook chapatis. A chapati cooked on a clay tawa is much more digestible than that cooked on a metal tawa, as it retains the nutrients. On the contrary, an aluminum tawa leaches metal particles into your body and leads toxic accumulation over time. Clay tawas are inexpensive and can easily be found in local Indian markets, or online.

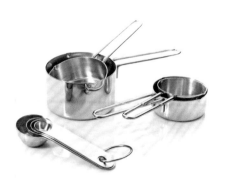

5. Measuring Cups and Spoons

While recreating recipes in this book, make sure you use the exact amount of the ingredients mentioned so that you get the perfect taste of the recipes. These are available on Amazon.

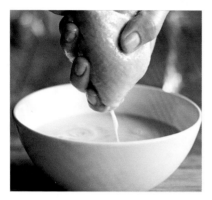

6. Nut Milk Bag *or* Muslin Cloth

A nut milk bag is basically a specially shaped fabric bag, that you strain your blended almond or coconut milk through, to remove any pulp that remains. A nut milk bag will help you achieve a smoother consistency of your coconut or almonds milks. This is available on Amazon. If you don't have a nut milk bag, a muslin cloth will work just fine.

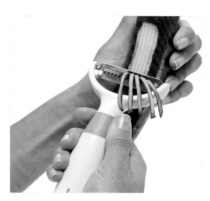

7. Julienne Vegetable Peeler

This is one seemingly gimmicky tool that I absolutely adore and highly recommend. A julienne peeler is a type of vegetable peeler with a jagged edge that allows you to create thin strips of vegetables for salads. Try it with zucchini, carrots, radish, cucumbers, beets, apples and more. Using this tool saves a lot of time and prevents fatigue while cutting vegetables for salads. This is available on Amazon.

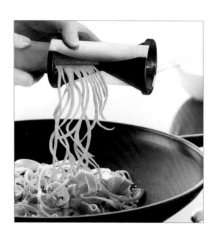

8. Spiraliser

A spiraliser is an inexpensive tool that turns fresh vegetables into noodles. As long as it's a hard fruit or veggie, you can spiralize it. Some great ones to spiralise are ridge gourd, bottle gourd, zucchini, beetroot, and cucumber. Spiralising is a sneaky way to eat more vegetables. "I'm eating spiralised noodles" is more exciting than saying "I'm eating a salad". This is available on Amazon.

How to use the tools?

1. How to use a *Julienne Vegetable Peeler*

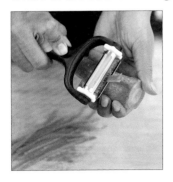 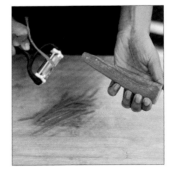 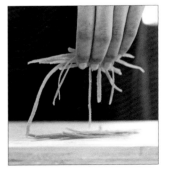

A. First, peel the vegetable with a standard peeler. Then, firmly hold the vegetable at an angle. Press the julienne peeler against the vegetable.

B. Peel the flesh, sliding the peeler away from you. Turn and repeat until you can no longer peel comfortably.

C. Using the julienne peeler, you can effortlessly create vegetable ribbons, and use them in salads or wraps.

2. How to use a *Spiraliser*

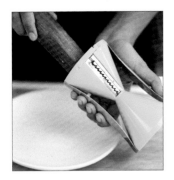 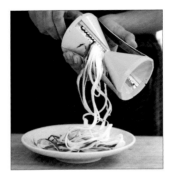 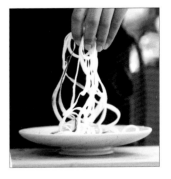

A. First, top and tail your vegetable and then insert it into the spiraliser. With most vegetables, you do not need to use the cap at this stage.

B. Twist the vegetable into the spiraliser (like a pencil sharpener). When you get near the bottom, use the cap (that comes with the spiraliser) so that you don't injure yourself.

C. A great dish to make with the resulting noodles is zucchini spaghetti.

41

Your body needs
Vegetable Sprouts

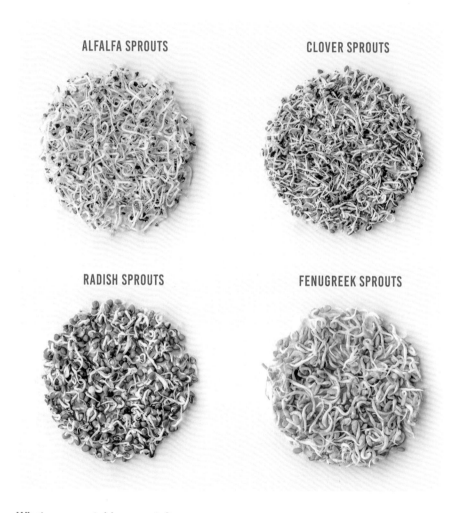

ALFALFA SPROUTS

CLOVER SPROUTS

RADISH SPROUTS

FENUGREEK SPROUTS

What are vegetable sprouts?

Vegetable sprouts are the most concentrated forms of living foods. When you soak and germinate seeds of vegetables, after 3-5 days, a white tail emerges from them. The seed, along with the tail are called vegetable sprouts. The easiest ones to grow in India are alfalfa, clover, radish and fenugreek.

Why Vegetable Sprouts?

Nutrition: Vegetable sprouts are one of the most nutritious whole foods on the planet. They are high-frequency, high-vibration living foods that transfers their life-force energy to you.

Cost Effective: Sprouted seeds multiply 3-15 times their weight. Grow organic food in your kitchen year round at a very minimal cost.

Organic: No chemicals, herbicide, pesticide or fungicide. You can trust that it's pure because you are the grower.

Easy: Just add water. No special lights required. You can grow half a kilo only in 9 square inches of counter space in your kitchen.

Freshness: Pick and eat the same day. No loss of nutrients.

Environment Friendly: No airplanes or fuel consumed to deliver this food to you

Emergency Preparedness: Sprout seeds last a long time if tightly sealed and stored in a cool, dry environment.

When you apply water to seeds, the seed absorbs the water and swells to at least twice its size. Not only does it swell in size, but it also swells in nutritional content. **Sprouts are 10 to 30 times more nutritious than the full grown vegetable.** They are plants in their baby stage. At this stage, they have the greatest concentration of nutrients than at any other point in their life. They are able to release these nutrients into our bodies because of their delicate cell walls.

This makes sprout a true "super food". They are one of the most LIVING FOODS in nature. Living foods are foods that create new life when planted. That small radish sprout has the life-force to grow a full-grown radish out of itself. This life-force is transferred to your body when you consume them. **Think about this, when you eat a sprout, you are eating the life-force energy that is needed to create a full grown healthy plant.**

Sprouts have been used as a health food throughout history. The Chinese have been using bean sprouts for centuries, since 3,000 BC to be exact, and swear by their healing properties. During world War II, sprouts were eaten as a source of protein.

Even Lord Jesus, in the Essene Gospel of Peace, recommends sprouting and explains how to make sprouted bread (also called Essene bread).

However, in India, people only know about lentil or bean sprouts. Barely anyone knows about vegetable sprouts. I learnt the concept of vegetable sprouts from Hippocrates Health Institute, where they are curing even third and fourth stage cancers by putting people on a raw food diet rich is vegetable sprouts.

Your body needs vegetable sprouts, not daal sprouts

Let's learn the difference between vegetable sprouts & daal sprouts.

Lentil & Bean Sprouts **Difficult to digest**	Vegetable Sprouts **Easy to digest**
Suitable only for athletes, children & manual laborers	Suitable for everyone
These are the varieties that we commonly recognize as sprouts. However, sprouts of beans & lentils are difficult to digest. They are ideal for children, athletes & people who do long hours of physical work. But they should be avoided by those trying to cure a disease or lose weight.	Some of the following varieties might seem new to you. Vegetables sprouts are much easier to digest than the sprouts of beans and grains.
Common varieties	Common varieties

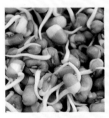
moong

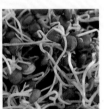
red lentils

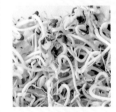
alfalfa

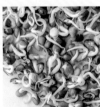
radish

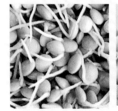
green lentils

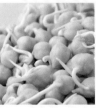
chickpea

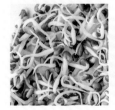
clover

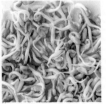
fenugreek

How to grow vegetable sprouts?

It's easy. Just 6 simple steps!

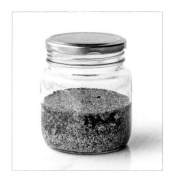

STEP 1 Rinse the seeds and place them in a glass container. Fill the container with filtered water to cover the seeds plus an inch. Let your seeds soak overnight.

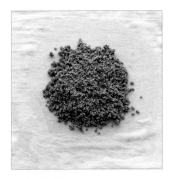

STEP 2 The following morning, drain out the water from the container. Rinse one time and drain again. Put your seeds at the center of the cotton cloth.

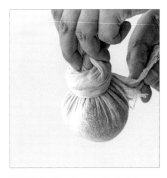

STEP 3 Tie the cloth tightly so that the seeds are contained in a bundle.

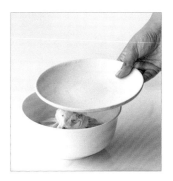

STEP 4 Place this bundle in a bowl and cover with plate. Make sure your cloth is not in direct sunlight.

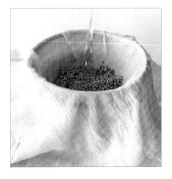

STEP 5 Rinse the seeds with fresh filtered water twice a day, one in the morning and once in the evening, for 4-5 days.

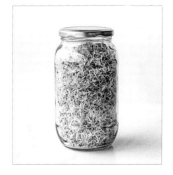

STEP 6 At the end of the rinsing time, your sprouts will be long enough to eat. The sprouting time will vary from seed to seed. Allow them to dry completely before storing. They can be stored in a covered container in the refrigerator for upto 5-7 days.

Sprouting Quantity Chart

Seed Type	Yield Amount	Rinsing Time
Alfalfa	1 tablespoon seeds = 1 cup sprouts	5 days
Clover	1 tablespoon seeds = 1 cup sprouts	5 days
Radish	2 tablespoon seeds = 1 cup sprouts	5 days
Fenugreek	1 tablespoon seeds = 1½ cups sprouts	3 days
Moong	½ cup seeds = 2 cup sprouts	3 days
Green Lentils	½ cup seeds = 2 cup sprouts	3 days

Sprouting FAQs

Where should I buy seeds?
You can order them online. They are also available on our website satvicmovement.org

Where should I store my seeds?
Keep them cool and dry. Seeds are often sold in plastic bags, which is fine if you plan on using them in a few months. If you plan in keeping them longer than that, transfer them to dry glass containers with a tight sealing lid. Store in pantry at room temperature. If it gets too hot, keep them in the refrigerator if you have space.

What is the best place to grow sprouts?
Your kitchen counter. The temperature, humidity, lighting, and proximity to a water source makes your kitchen an ideal setting to grow your sprouts.

What is the best temperature?
Between 17-22 degrees C (65 and 75 degrees F).

How much light does it need?
Not much. You can keep them on your kitchen counter. You never want any direct sunlight hitting your sprouts, otherwise, they will get too hot, cook and die.

What kind of water should I use?
Filtered water at room temperature.

Where should I store my sprouts?
In the refrigerator in a covered container. Make sure they are completely dry before you store them. They should last for 5-7 days.

What if the sprouts develop mold?
Increase ventilation around your jars. A ceiling or tabletop fan on "low" somewhere in the room is ideal.

How to use vegetable sprouts?

Sprouts are great to use in salads because they instantly add crunchiness, flavor and nutrition to your meal. To make a fulfilling salad, use 30% sprouts, 30% vegetables, 30% leafy greens and 10% toppings, such as coconut, nuts, seeds, homemade dressings (for the sake of taste and texture).

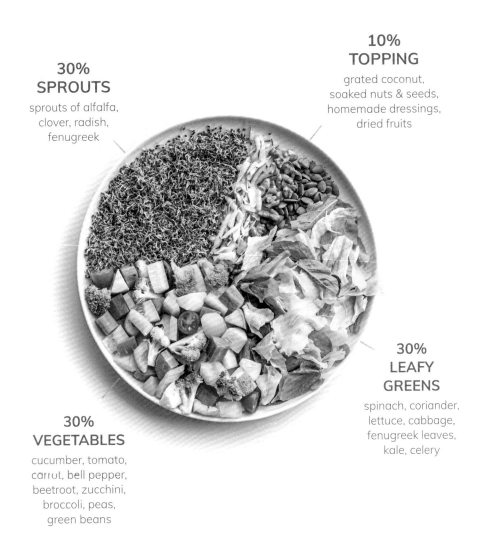

**10%
TOPPING**
grated coconut,
soaked nuts & seeds,
homemade dressings,
dried fruits

**30%
SPROUTS**
sprouts of alfalfa,
clover, radish,
fenugreek

**30%
LEAFY
GREENS**
spinach, coriander,
lettuce, cabbage,
fenugreek leaves,
kale, celery

**30%
VEGETABLES**
cucumber, tomato,
carrot, bell pepper,
beetroot, zucchini,
broccoli, peas,
green beans

All about nut milks

Nut Milk refers to non-dairy milks derived from plants or nuts, such as coconuts, almonds, hazelnuts, cashews or sunflower seeds. As you keep following this lifestyle, nut milks will become a staple in your kitchen.

How are nut milks made?
Nut milks are made from different types of nuts. First, nuts are soaked in water for 6-8 hours. Then, they are blended together with fresh water. The liquid that is strained from this mixture is the nut milk. In some cases, natural flavoring (for example - dates, cinnamon, etc) is added.

Which is healthiest nut milk?
Coconut milk. Coconut is easier to digest than any other nut milk.

How can I use nut milks?
Nut milks can be used as bases for smoothies, soups, curries, dressings and desserts.

How often can I consume them?
Most recipes in this book already include coconut milk. There is no need to drink nut milk separately. Nut milks are heavy.

Can I buy pre-packaged nut milks?
No. They are chock-full of preservative, thickeners, and artificial ingredients.

Note
- Use only raw and un-fried nuts, strictly no roasted nuts.
- Nuts must be soaked for at least 5-6 hours in fresh water. In case you are in a hurry, soak them in hot water for about 30 minutes.
- Always discard the water in which the nuts had been soaked.
- Do not make soy milk as it very difficult to digest.
- Make sure you never cook coconut milk directly on flame. Coconut milk is extremely nutritious but when cooked, it converts into cholesterol. Always add it towards the end after switching off the stove.

How to make coconut milk?

MAKES 2 CUPS

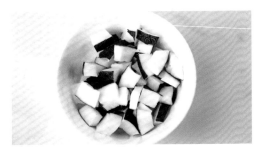

1. Take 1 cup of fresh dessicated coconut.

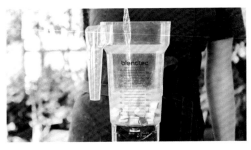

2. Combine it with 2 cups of water in a blender.

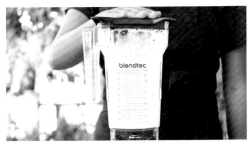

3. Blend until smooth.

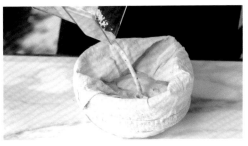

4. Pour the mixture over a bowl covered with a nut milk bag or a muslin cloth.

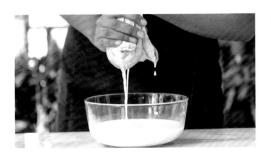

5. Squeeze out the milk with your hand. You can use the leftover pulp as a face scrub.

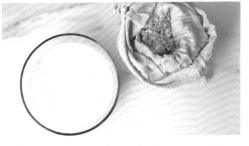

6. Milk can be used immediately or stored in refrigerator for upto 1-2 days.

FOR MAKING ALMOND MILK,

Replace 1 cup dessicated coconut with 1 cup almonds, soaked in water for 5-6 hours.

DO's and DONT's
of recipe making

1. Use exact measurements

Please use the exact measurements of the ingredients mentioned in the recipes, in order to get the right taste of the dishes. We often see people casually adding ingredients, without measuring them with measuring cups and spoons and as a result, they do not get the desired taste, consistency or texture. After a few months of following the Satvic recipes, you might remember the measurements, but please carefully measure the ingredients in the beginning.

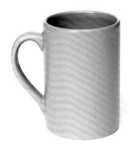

DON'T USE THIS ✖

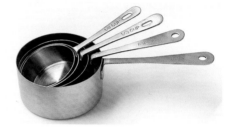

USE THIS ✓

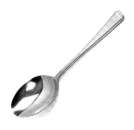

DON'T USE THIS ✖

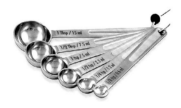

USE THIS ✓

2. *If making conversions, follow the conversion chart below*

   ¼ cup = 4 tablespoons
   ½ cup = 8 tablespoons
   1 tablespoon = 3 teaspoons
   1 pinch = 1/16 teaspoon

3. *When using dry herbs, use less.* Dry herbs are more concentrated. It's a 1:3 ratio. If using 1 tablespoon of fresh, use 1 teaspoon of dry.

4. Always **soak your seeds** in water before using. Nuts contain something called enzyme inhibitors, which make them hard to digest. By soaking them, these enzyme inhibitors are removed. The average soak time for nuts is 6 hours. You may soak them overnight.

5. *For maximum health value, please stick to the recipes exactly.* Do not increase the amount of grains, nuts or spices in a dish. The recipes have been created keeping in mind strict food principles to ensure fastest healing and maximum health.

CHAPTER 3
SATVIC
MEAL PLANS

It is not enough to eat some Satvic food every now and then. To see real results, you must bring a total shift in your diet & lifestyle. You must religiously follow the meal plan presented on the next page.

Choose your meal plan

Given below are four different meal plans.

The **happy disease plan** is for times you need to fast (eat no solid food). It should be followed in case of an acute disease - such as fever, cold, cough, headache, sore throat, vomiting , diarrhoea or any acute pain.

The healing plan is for those trying to reverse a chronic disease or lose weight. If you are suffering from diabetes, thyroid imbalance, PCOD, hypertension, sinusitis, asthma, cysts, stones, chronic gastritis/acidity, chronic constipation, skin problems, hair problems, joint or bone problems or any other chronic disease, please follow the healing plan. In this plan, one should eat grains not more than once a day.

The **lifestyle plan** is for those who have no disease and are wanting to maintain their health. After reversing your health problems completely, you may switch to the lifestyle plan.

The building plan is for children below age 16 (if not suffering from any health problem), people engaged in heavy physical exercise (more than 3 hours everyday), pregnant women (if not suffering from any health problem) and those wanting to gain weight (if not suffering from any health problem). In such cases, one can eat grains twice a day.

Please Note -

- You may swap lunch and dinner in any of the plans if that is more convenient for you.

- You can adjust the timings mentioned in the meal plans according to your schedule. However, always follow 16 hour fasting between your dinner and breakfast, to give your body a chance to rest and repair every night.

- Those in the building plan can do 14 hour fasting instead of 16 hour fasting.

- The recipes in this book have been structured according to the healing plan, as it is suited to most people reading this book.

	Building	Lifestyle	Healing	Happy Disease
Recommended for :	• Children below 16 (if healthy) • Those doing more than 3 hrs of intense exercise everyday • Pregnant women (if healthy) • Those wanting to gain weight (if healthy)	Those wanting to maintain their health. No current disease	• Those wanting to reverse a chronic disease • Those wanting to lose weight	Fever, cold, cough, headache, sore throat, vomiting, diarrhoea, or any other acute disease
Pre-Breakfast 8:00 am	**Nourishing Juice** any fresh seasonal fruit juice (for example juice of watermelon, orange, pomegranate) or ABC Juice	**Detox Juice** Ash gourd juice or coconut water or vegetable juice	**Detox Juice** Ash gourd juice or coconut water or vegetable juice	**Detox Juice** Ash gourd juice or coconut water or vegetable juice
Breakfast 10:00 am	**Smoothie or smoothie bowl** using dense fruits such as banana, mango or chikoo with nuts, seeds and dates.	**Seasonal Fruits or Smoothie or Smoothie Bowl**	**Mono Fruit** Any one seasonal fruit	**Detox Juice** Ash gourd juice or coconut water or vegetable juice
Lunch 1:00 pm	**Pulse Meal** any one pulse (such as chickpea, lentils, kidney beans) with lots of veggies	**Grain Meal** satvic roti-sabzi or any grain with lots of veggies	**Grain Meal** satvic roti-sabzi or any grain with lots of veggies	**Detox Juice** Ash gourd juice or coconut water or vegetable juice
Mid-Meal 4:00 pm	**Seasonal Fruits or Smoothie or Coconut Water**	3-5 dates with 4-5 pcs of coconut giri or a handful of soaked nuts or bowl of vegetable sprouts	—	
Dinner 6:00 pm	**Grain Meal** satvic roti-sabzi or any grain with lots of veggies	**Satvic Salad** with nut or seed based dressing or **Satvic Soup** with steamed vegetables	**Satvic Salad or Satvic Soup**	**Vegetable Broth**

CHAPTER 4

RECIPES FOR THE REVOLUTION

Following is a collection of recipes complying to all 21 Satvic food principles. There are soups, salads, smoothies, juices, main meals and different cuisines including Indian, South Indian, Thai & Italian. We hope you have fun on this exciting new journey of vitality, health & happiness.

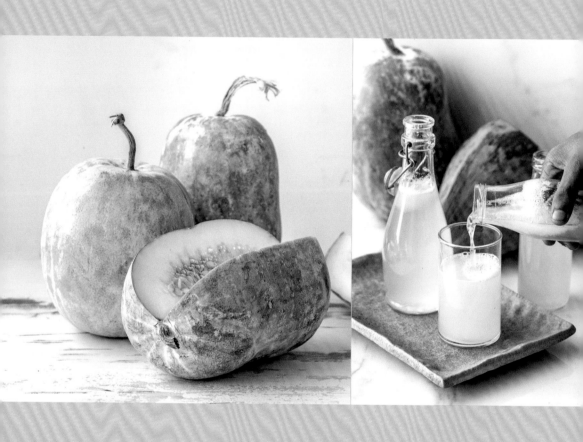

1st meal
PRE-BREAKFAST

Always start your day with something light and detoxifying. When we start a car, we don't immediately set it on fifth gear. We start with first gear and gradually move upto the fifth gear. Same with our body. We should start our day with a detox juice. Then eat fruits for breakfast, a grain meal for lunch & finish with a light dinner.

PRE-BREAKFAST

Pre-breakfast is basically your morning detox juice. You can have this 1-2 hours after waking up. Make sure to maintain a gap of 2 hours between pre-breakfast and breakfast. When you drink a detox juice, it starts doing it's work inside, that is, it starts cleaning your body. If you eat something immediately after the detox juice, the cleaning gets interrupted.

Below are the three options we suggest for pre-breakfast.

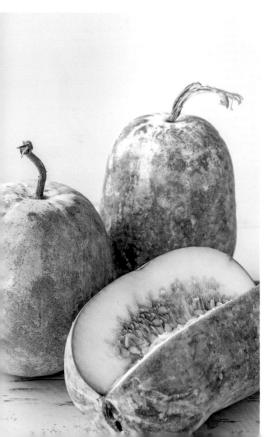

1st option (best option)

ASH GOURD JUICE

Ash gourd *(safed petha)* is one of the most detoxifying vegetables in Nature. When it enters our body, it starts to suck in all the toxins and when it leaves our body, it carries with it all the toxic waste. It is like a sponge in our digestive system. Many people tell that their stomach immediately gets cleared after drinking ash gourd juice.

Ash Gourd is easy to find at vegetable vendors. It belongs to the gourd family and is also called 'winter melon'. Don't worry, the taste of ash gourd juice is not bitter at all. In fact, it's quite bland, like water.

INGREDIENTS
Ash gourd *(safed petha)*

METHOD
1. Remove the peel of the ash gourd and take out all the seeds from inside.
2. Cut it into pieces and juice it. Drink about 400 ml (1 glass) of this juice every morning.

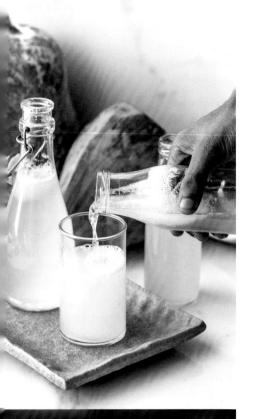

2nd best option

ASH COCO JUICE

If for some reason you do not like the taste of ash gourd, or want to give it to children, you may mix the ash gourd juice with 50% coconut water.

INGREDIENTS

50% ash gourd juice
50% coconut water

METHOD

1. Mix the ash gourd juice with 50% coconut water.
2. Drink about 400 ml (1 glass) of this ash coco juice every morning.

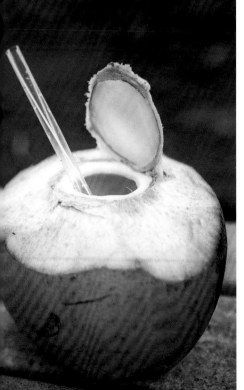

3rd best option

COCONUT WATER

Coconut is called "*Shree Phal*" in Sanskrit. It's the only fruit which is given the title *Shree* in front of it, because of it's healing properties. Coconut water is a natural laxative. Make sure you only use fresh coconut water, not the pre-packaged or bottled version. In case coconut water is not available in your country, you can drink the juice of any other fresh green vegetable - such as celery, cucumber, bottle gourd, spinach, etc.

INGREDIENTS

400 ml (about 1 glass) of coconut water

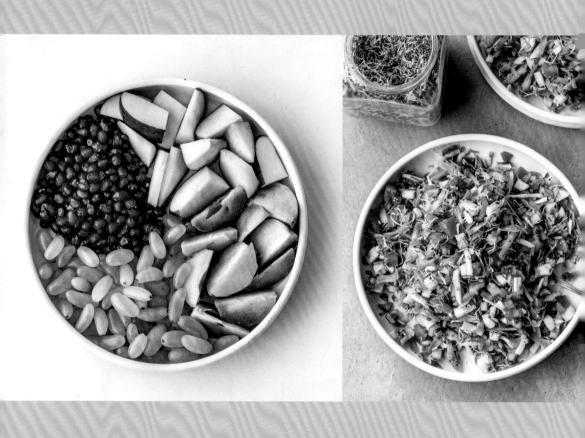

2nd meal

BREAKFAST

For maximum energy throughout the day, you should eat a light breakfast, consisting of water-rich fruits or a pure Satvic salad. The philosophy of eating a heavy breakfast (recently brought about by the Western influence) is highly flawed. This culture came about food companies that wanted to sell cereal boxes. In the morning, our stomach is still busy digesting the last bits of our dinner. If we eat a heavy breakfast, the body shifts its energy to address the new food. The undigested dinner results in the production of waste, or, toxins in the body.

BREAKFAST

BREAKFAST

You should have your breakfast 2 hours after your morning detox juice (pre-breakfast). For breakfast, you can either have fresh fruits, a smoothie or the pure Satvic salad.

If you have fruits for breakfast, have salad for dinner. If you eat salad for breakfast, you may have fruits for dinner. It is important to maintain a balance between eating fruits and vegetables.

If you have diabetes, avoid sweet fruits (such as mango, pineapple, *chikoo*, banana) and stick to neutral fruits (such as melon and papaya).

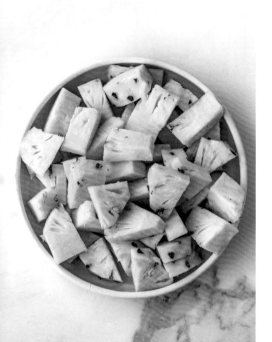

1st option

EATING 1 FRUIT AT A TIME

It is best to eat only 1 type of fruit at a time. This is called 'mono-eating'. It is easier for our stomach to digest 1 fruit, rather than many fruits, as each fruit requires a different type of digestive juice to be secreted by the stomach.

You can eat a plate full of any seasonal fruit, for example :

- melons (such as watermelon or muskmelon)
- apple
- pear
- pineapple
- orange
- papaya
- peach
- pomegranate
- berries
- guava

Just make sure whatever you eat is seasonal & regional. Do not eat fruits imported from other countries.

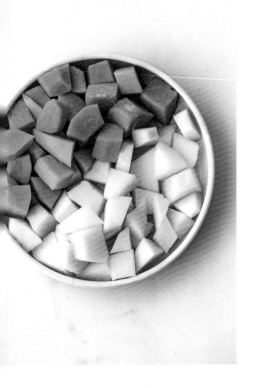

EATING 2 FRUITS

If you feel bored of eating only 1 fruit, you may eat two fruits together. If possible, mix same categories of fruits together. Below are points to keep in mind from the digestive point of view :

- mix melons only with melons
- do not mix sweet fruits (such as mango, chikoo) with citric fruits (such as oranges, pineapple, kiwi)

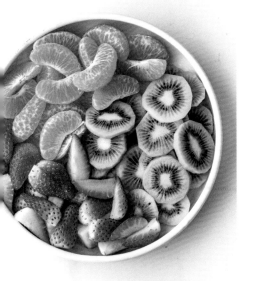

3rd option

EATING 2 OR MORE FRUITS

If you feel bored eating only 2 fruits, you may eat more than 2 fruits. It is not bad, but it is slower to digest compared to eating only one fruit at a time. Even when eating multiple fruits, try to mix only the same categories of fruits together. Do not mix citrus and sweet.

BREAKFAST

SMOOTHIES

Occasionally, you may replace your fruit bowls with a smoothie. A smoothie with banana, coconut milk or dry fruits is heavier to digest than eating fruits alone. Hence, we suggest having it only occasionally in the healing stage. For those who are doing vigorous exercise and for children, it is quite good. To build a delicious smoothie, you need 4 components-

1. **Liquid component** - Coconut milk, coconut water, watery fruits or drinking water
2. **Base** - Any fruit or vegetable such as banana, pear, melon, papaya, beetroot, carrots, spinach, lettuce, etc.
3. **Sweetener** - Sweet fruits such as mangoes, banana or dates.
4. **Flavor** - Herbs such as mint or basil, carob powder, cacao powder, vanilla powder, ginger, etc.

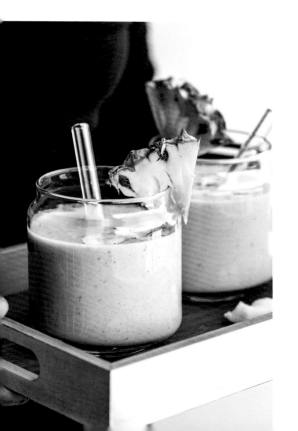

PIÑA COLADA SMOOTHIE

INGREDIENTS
SERVES 1, MAKES 500 ML

- 1 cup pineapple chunks
- 1 cup coconut milk
- ½ medium banana
- ¼ cup ice cubes
- 2 dates, seedless
- ⅛ teaspoon vanilla bean powder (optional)

METHOD

1. Place everything into a blender and blend until smooth. Serve.

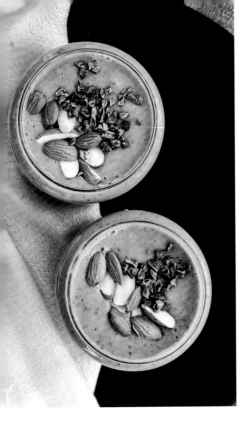

Drink as an occasional treat!

BANANA DATE SHAKE

INGREDIENTS
SERVES 2, MAKES 700 ML

- 1½ cups coconut milk
- 3 bananas
- 6 dates, seedless
- 4 ice cubes
- ½ teaspoon cinnamon powder

METHOD

1. Place coconut milk, bananas, dates, ice and cinnamon into a blender and blend until smooth Serve.

TROPICAL SMOOTHIE

INGREDIENTS
SERVES 1, MAKES 500 ML

- 1 cup coconut water
- 1 cup chopped spinach
- 1 cup chopped apple
- 1 cup mango chunks
- ½ teaspoon lemon juice

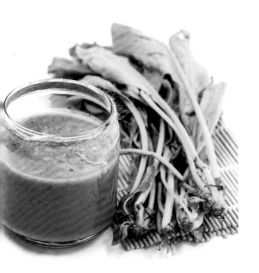

METHOD

1. Place all the ingredients into a blender and blend until smooth.
2. Let the smoothie cool in the refrigerator for about 20 minutes before serving.

Substitution : If mango is out of season, replace it with 1 cup chopped guava & 2 seedless dates.

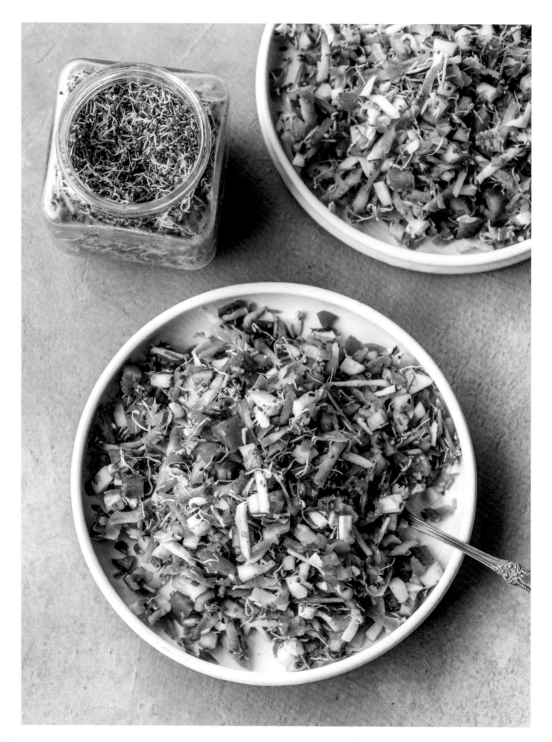

PURE SATVIC SALAD

BEST FOR

○ Morning Detox Drink ✓ Lunch ✓ Dinner
✓ Breakfast ○ Mid-Meal ○ An Occasional Treat

This salad is called the pure Satvic salad because it is the purest and cleanest salad amongst the other salads in this book. It does not contain any nuts, seeds, dressings, salt or lemon because ideally, a salad should be eaten with no condiments at all. Yet, this salad is flavorful (because of the coriander and coconut) and crunchy (because of the sprouts).

INGREDIENTS
SERVES 2

- 2 cucumbers, chopped
- 2 carrots, grated
- 2 tomatoes, chopped
- 1 small green capsicum, chopped
- 1 cup coriander, chopped
- 2 big slices of coconut, grated

For a boost
- ½ cup vegetable sprouts (such as alfalfa, clover, radish, fenugreek).

PRE-PREPARATION

(optional) Prepare vegetable sprouts as explained on page 42.

METHOD

1. Place all the ingredients into a large mixing bowl. Toss everything together and serve.

Note Make sure you use vegetable sprouts in this salad, not lentil sprouts. Lentil sprouts should only be consumed by athletes or children, as they are harder to digest.

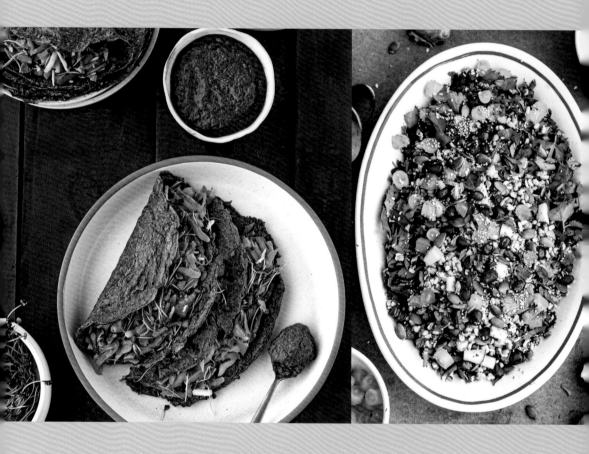

LUNCH

Our digestive power is the highest during noon and hence, we recommend that you eat you eat your grain meal (heaviest meal of the day) during this time. On the following pages, there are grain recipes that you may have for lunch. Please remember the points below -

1. Eat only one type of grain at a time. Do not mix more than one grain in the same meal. So no chapati with rice, no rice with cheelas, no daliya with quinoa.
2. Eat less grain & more vegetable. If you eat one bowl of grain, eat 3 bowls of vegetable.
3. After your lunch, take rest for 20 minutes, so that your energy gets fully diverted to digesting your food.
4. If you wish you can also eat your grain meal for dinner and soup/salad meal for lunch.

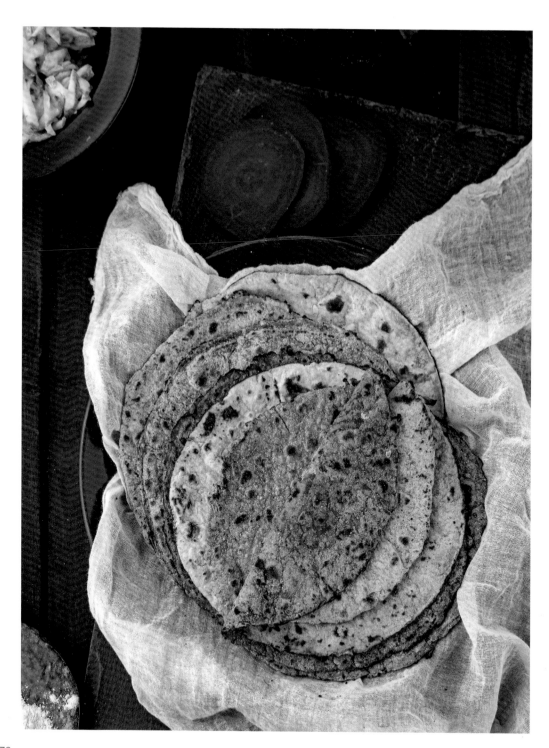

COMPOSITE CHAPATI

INGREDIENTS

- 50% wheat flour
- 50% any seasonal vegetable (such as cucumber, bottle gourd, beetroot, carrot, spinach, fenugreek (*methi*) leaves, coriander, pumpkin, ridge gourd (*tori*), ash gourd).

METHOD

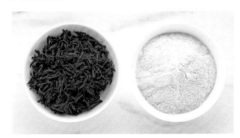

STEP 1 Take one cup of any seasonal vegetable (grated) & one cup of wheat flour.

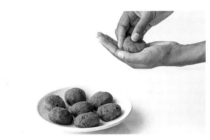

STEP 2 Combine them together. Use water if required. Make a dough & divide it into balls. Dip the balls in flour and flatten them.

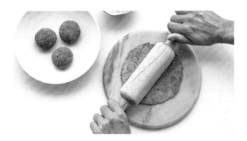

STEP 3 Roll the balls with a rolling pin.

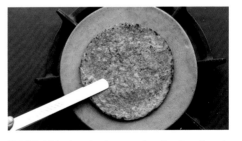

STEP 4 Heat a clay tawa on low heat and cook the chapati on it. Do not use oil or ghee.

Scan to watch
the video

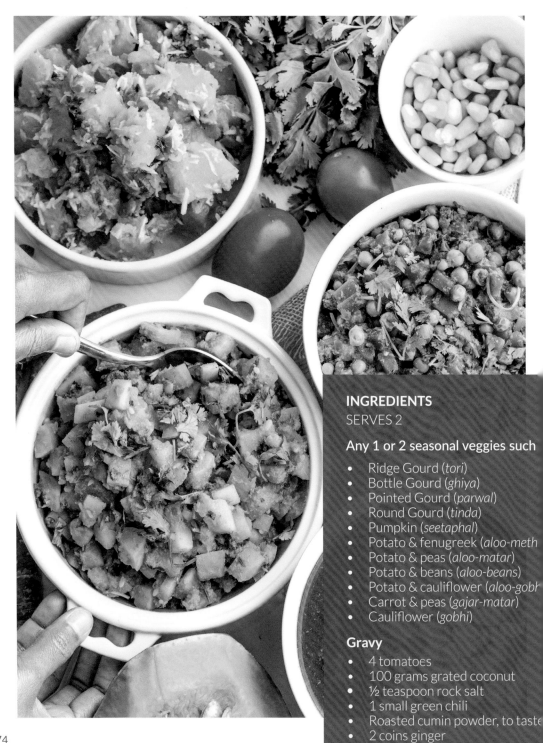

INGREDIENTS
SERVES 2

Any 1 or 2 seasonal veggies such

- Ridge Gourd (*tori*)
- Bottle Gourd (*ghiya*)
- Pointed Gourd (*parwal*)
- Round Gourd (*tinda*)
- Pumpkin (*seetaphal*)
- Potato & fenugreek (*aloo-meth*
- Potato & peas (*aloo-matar*)
- Potato & beans (*aloo-beans*)
- Potato & cauliflower (*aloo-gobh*
- Carrot & peas (*gajar-matar*)
- Cauliflower (*gobhi*)

Gravy

- 4 tomatoes
- 100 grams grated coconut
- ½ teaspoon rock salt
- 1 small green chili
- Roasted cumin powder, to taste
- 2 coins ginger

SATVIC SABZI

METHOD

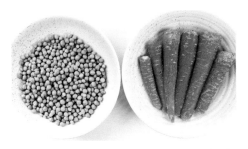 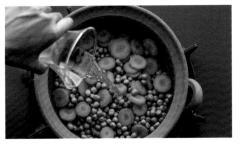

1. Take any 1 or 2 seasonal vegetables. Soak in water for about 2 hours to reduce the impact of chemicals in the vegetables.

2. Peel & chop the vegetables. Add to a clay pot along with some water. Close the lid and let them cook in water until soft.

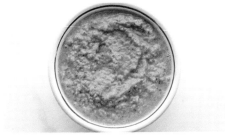 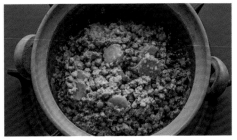

3. Meanwhile, prepare the gravy. Blend together tomatoes, coconut, salt, chili, cumin and ginger until smooth.

4. Combine gravy with boiled vegetables. Close the lid, switch off the stove & let the gravy cook through the steam inside the pot for 10 minutes. Top with coriander & serve.

Note Do not re-heat sabzi after adding gravy. Coconut & tomatoes should never be cooked directly on the flame. .

Scan to watch
the video

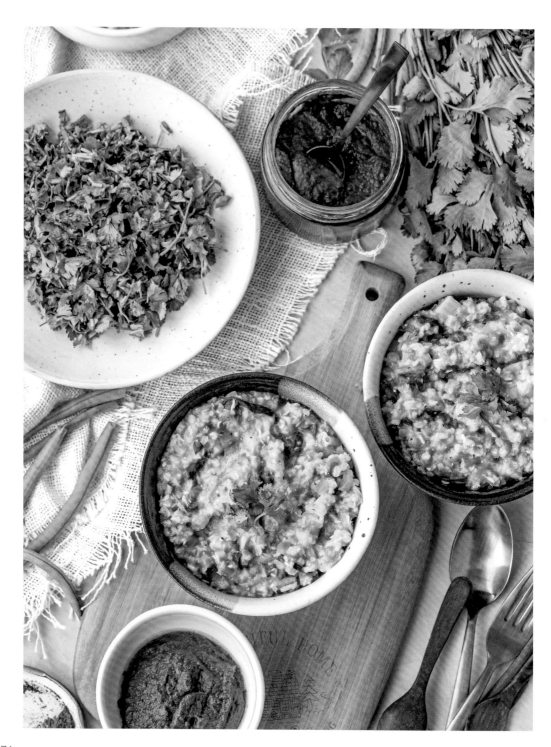

SATVIC KHICHADI

BEST FOR

○ Morning Detox Drink   ☑ Lunch   ○ Dinner
○ Breakfast   ○ Mid-Meal   ○ An Occasional Treat

The commonly made khichadi with lots of daal, rice, spices and oil is difficult to digest if you're living a sedentary lifestyle. It has few vegetables and lots of grains which makes is heavy. In Satvic khichadi, if we use 1 cup of rice, we use four times more vegetables. Why? Because adding a sufficiency of vegetables to the grain makes the grain easier to digest.

LUNCH

INGREDIENTS
SERVES 3

- 1 cup soaked brown rice
- 6 cups water
- 1 cup finely chopped green beans
- 1 cup grated carrot
- 1 cup grated bottle guard
- 1 teaspoon turmeric powder
- 1 cup finely chopped spinach
- 2 small green chillies, finely crushed
- 1 cup chopped tomato
- ½ cup coconut kernel, sliced and then blended in a blender
- 2 teaspoons rock salt
- ½ cup chopped coriander

Green Chutney (pg 90)

PRE-PREPARATION

Soak brown rice in water for about 3 hours.

METHOD

1. In a pot, place the brown rice along with 6 cups of water. Let it cook on a low flame till it turns soft (about 45 minutes). Keep stirring in between.

2. Add the beans, carrots, bottle guard and turmeric and cook for another 15 minutes. Add more water if required.

3. Add the spinach and green chillies. Stir well and cook for another 5 minutes.

4. Turn off the stove. Add the tomatoes, coconut and salt. Keep the pot covered for 5 minutes.

5. Top with coriander and serve with green chutney.

Scan to watch
the video

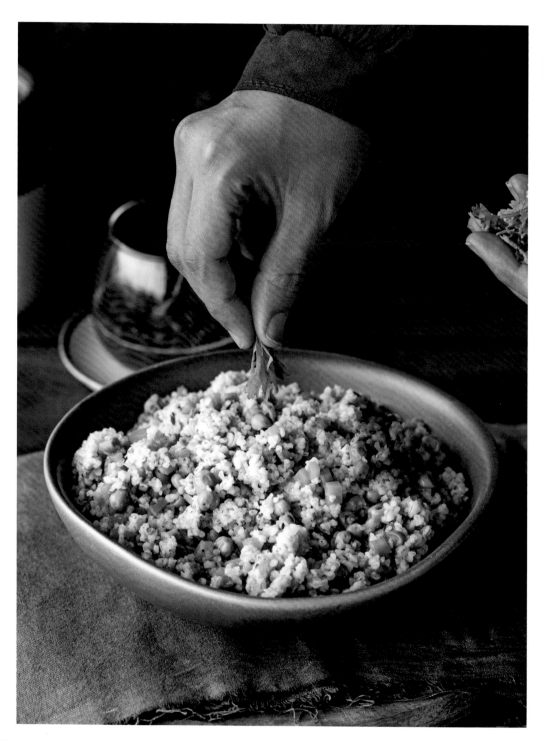

SATVIC DALIYA

BEST FOR

- ○ Morning Detox Drink
- ○ Breakfast
- ✓ Lunch
- ○ Mid-Meal
- ○ Dinner
- ○ An Occasional Treat

The Satvic Daliya uses less grain and more vegetables. The ratio is 1:3 (1 cup grain to 3 cups vegetables). Why? Because grains are hard to digest. Our body has to spend a lot of time processing grains (about 18 hours). But when combined with vegetables, less grain goes inside the body, so it can spend less time digesting and more time healing itself.

LUNCH

INGREDIENTS
SERVES 2-3

- 1 cup broken wheat porridge (*daliya*)
- 1½ teaspoons cumin seeds
- 1 cup green beans, finely chopped
- 1 cup carrots, finely chopped
- 1 cup green peas
- 2 small green chilies, very finely crushed
- 4 cups water
- 2 teaspoons rock salt
- Handful fresh coriander

Green Chutney (pg 90)

METHOD

1. Roast the broken wheat porridge lightly in a pan till it turns light brown. Then, take it out in a bowl.

2. Take another pan. Heat it on a medium flame. Add the cumin seeds and roast till they are dark brown. Add the beans, carrots and peas and stir well. Add the finely crushed green chilies and stir again.

3. Add 4 cups of water to the pan and let it come to a boil. Then, add the roasted porridge to the pan. Cover the pan and keep the stove on a medium flame till the porridge absorbs all the water.

4. Once everything is cooked, turn off the stove. Add rock salt and keep it covered for 5 minutes.

5. Garnish with generous amounts of fresh coriander and enjoy with green chutney. Eat within 3-4 hours of preparing it.

Scan to watch the video

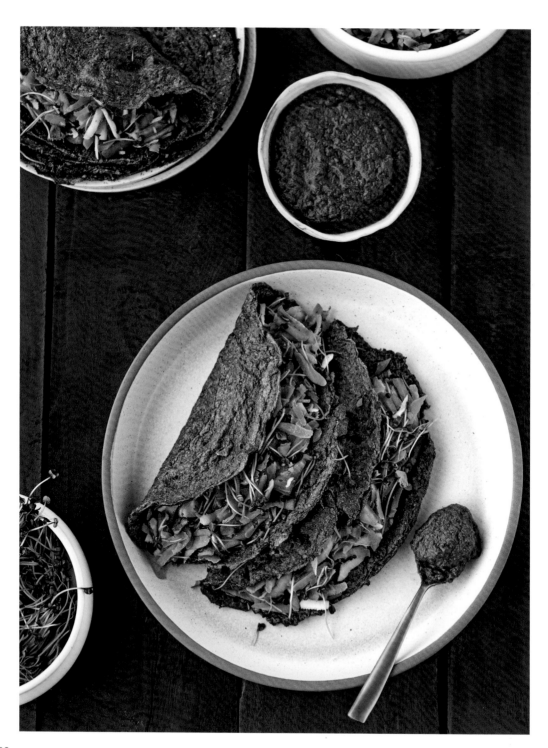

SPINACH CHEELA

BEST FOR

○ Morning Detox Drink
○ Breakfast

✓ Lunch
○ Mid-Meal

○ Dinner
○ An Occasional Treat

In Satvic Cheela, instead of using only lentils, we use 50% lentils and 50% spinach. Why? because lentils are difficult to digest for people living a sedentary lifestyle. Unless you're an athlete or a child in the growing stage, you should eat lentils sparingly.

INGREDIENTS
MAKES 8-10 CHEELAS

For the Cheelas
- 1 cup green split moong daal
- 1 teaspoon rock salt
- 1 small green chili, chopped
- 2 cups spinach purée*

For the Filling
- 4 carrots, thickly grated and lightly steamed
- 4 tomatoes, chopped finely
- ½ cup grated coconut
- ½ cup coriander, chopped
- 1 teaspoon rock salt

Green Chutney (pg 90)

*2 ½ cups of chopped spinach, when blended, gives 2 cups of spinach puree.

PRE-PREPARATION
Soak moong daal in water for about 3 hours.

METHOD

1. Combine the soaked moong daal, salt and chili in a blender and blend until smooth. Transfer the mixture to a bowl. Add the spinach puree to the mixture and stir well.

2. Heat an iron pan (tava), sprinkle a little water on it and wipe it off gently using a muslin cloth. Pour a ladle full of the batter on it and spread it in a circular motion to make a thin circle. Cook on a medium flame till it turns brownish-green.

3. To prepare the filling, simply combine the lightly steamed carrots, tomatoes, coconut, coriander, microgreens and salt. Fill your cheelas with this filling, and serve immediately with green chutney.

LUNCH

Scan to watch
the video

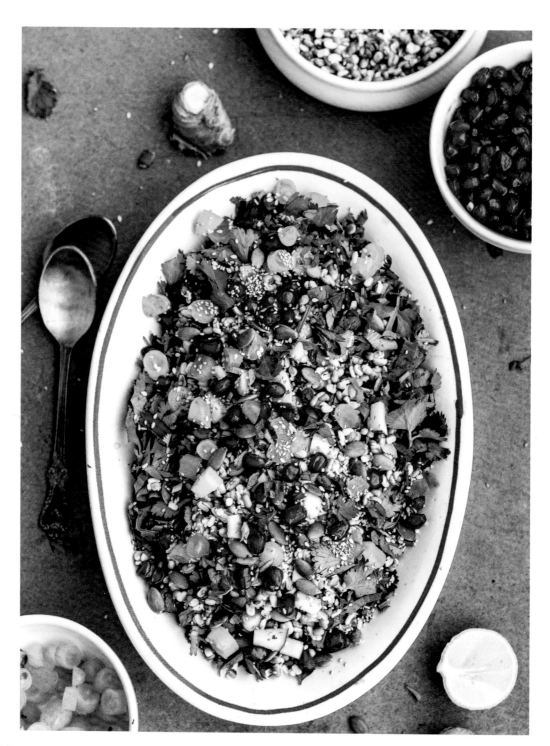

MOONG BOWL

BEST FOR

- ○ Morning Detox Drink
- ○ Breakfast
- ✔ Lunch
- ○ Mid-Meal
- ○ Dinner
- ○ An Occasional Treat

A refreshing bowl which is fully raw. No ingredient in this recipe has been heated or cooked, thus preserving all the nutrition in the ingredients. It's easy to make and hence a great option when you don't have much time to cook.

INGREDIENTS
SERVES 3

- ½ cup split moong daal with skin
- 1½ cup finely chopped fresh fenugreek (*methi*) leaves
- 1 cup finely chopped coriander
- 1½ cup diced apple
- 1½ cup chopped grapes
- 1½ cup pomegranate
- 2 tablespoons chia seeds
- 2 tablespoons pumpkin seeds
- 2 tablespoons white sesame seeds

Flavoring
- 1 teaspoon grated fresh ginger
- 2 tablespoons lemon juice
- 1 teaspoon rock salt
- 1 green chili, crushed
- ⅛ teaspoon asafoetida (*hing*)

PRE-PREPARATION

Soak split moong daal in water for about 4 hours.

METHOD

1. Place the moong daal, methi, coriander, apple, grapes, pomegranate, chia seeds, pumpkin seeds and sesame seeds into a large mixing bowl. Mix well.

2. Place all the flavoring ingredients into a small mixing bowl and mix well, so they become infused together.

3. Add this flavoring to the rest of the ingredients, mix well and serve.

LUNCH

Scan to watch the video

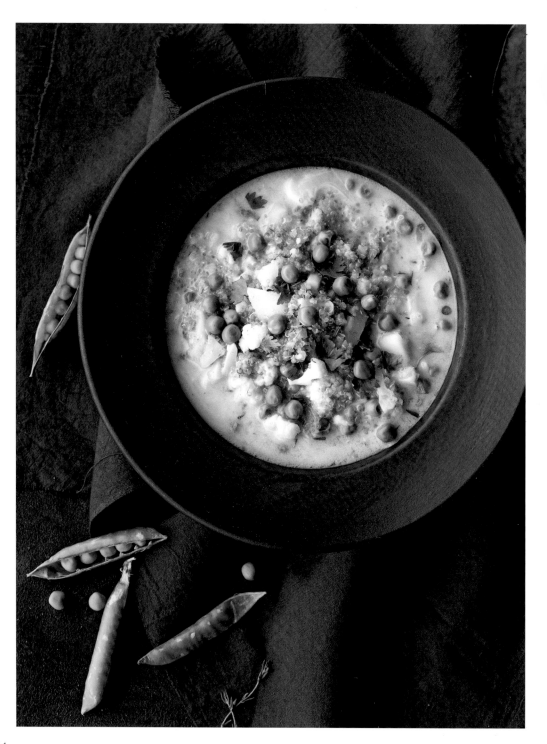

COCO QUINOA BOWL

BEST FOR

○ Morning Detox Drink ☑ Lunch ○ Dinner
○ Breakfast ○ Mid-Meal ○ An Occasional Treat

Technically, quinoa is a seed, but we classify it under the umbrella of 'grains' because it has the same digestibility level as grains. This recipe is delicious. The herbs - thyme and coriander come together to create an exquisite flavor.

INGREDIENTS
SERVES 2-3

- 1 cup quinoa
- 3 ½ cups water
- 1 cup green peas
- 3 cups chopped cauliflower
- 2 small potatoes, diced
- 1 teaspoon ginger, grated
- 1 teaspoon green chili, crushed
- 1 tablespoon fresh thyme or 1 teaspoon dried thyme
- 2 cups coconut milk
- 2 ½ teaspoons rock salt
- 1 tablespoon lemon juice
- ½ cup chopped coriander

PRE-PREPARATION

Prepare coconut milk.

METHOD

1. Wash the quinoa. Place it in a saucepan along with 2½ cups water & let it cook on low flame till the quinoa absorbs the water. Add more water if necessary.

2. In another saucepan, add 1 cup of water along with the peas, cauliflower and potatoes and cook till soft to bite. Then, take out all the vegetables from the pan and store the broth aside.

3. Add the vegetables to the quinoa. Stir well.

4. Add ginger, chili and thyme and stir for ½ a minute.

5. Switch off the stove & add coconut milk, salt & lemon. Cover the pan for 5 minutes so the ingredients cook in the steam inside, not directly on the flame.

6. Top with coriander, stir well and serve immediately.

Scan to watch
the video

LUNCH

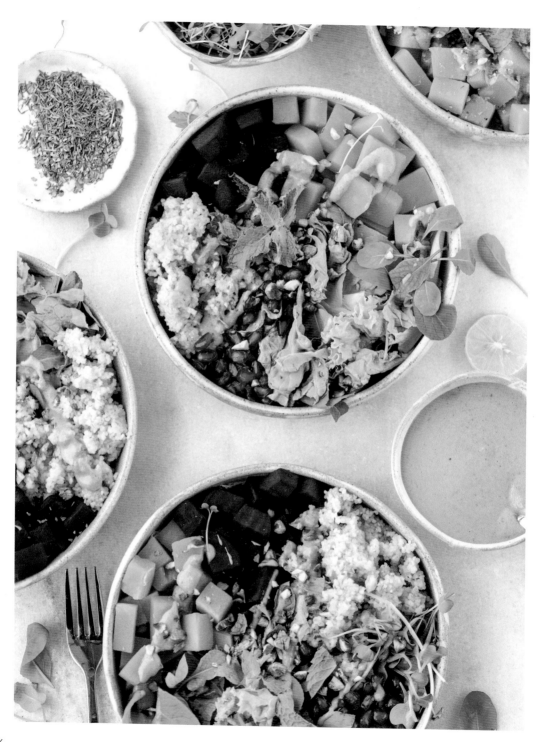

BARLEY BOWL

BEST FOR

○ Morning Detox Drink ☑ Lunch ○ Dinner
○ Breakfast ○ Mid-Meal ○ An Occasional Treat

INGREDIENTS

SERVES 3

- ¼ cup barley dalia seeds
- 1 cup torn lettuce leaves
- ¾ cup torn spinach leaves
- 1 cup chopped pumpkin
- 1 cup chopped beetroot
- 1 tablespoon lemon juice
- 1 tablespoon dried thyme
- 1 teaspoon dried oregano
- 1 teaspoon rock salt
- ½ cup pomegranate

Mint Tahini Dressing

- 3 tablespoons homemade tahini
- 1 tablespoon lemon juice
- ½ teaspoon rock salt
- 1 inch green chilli
- ¼ cup mint leaves
- ¼ cup water

Topping

- ⅛ cup mint leaves, finely chopped
- 1 tablespoon crushed pistachios

METHOD

1. Boil the ¼ cup barley seeds with ½ cup water until all the water is absorbed and barley dalia is cooked.

2. Steam the pumpkin and beetroot till soft.

3. Add the lemon juice, thyme, oregano & salt to the steamed pumpkin and beetroot.

4. Mix the pomegranate with the cooked barley dalia.

5. To make the **mint tahini dressing**, blend all ingredients of the dressing until smooth.

6. Mix the mint tahini dressing with the lettuce and spinach using a spatula.

7. In a serve bowling, serve the three components of the bowl separately i.e. the green leafy vegetables, the beetroot-pumpkin and the barley dalia.

8. Top with mint leaves and crushed pistachio and serve.

Scan to watch
the video

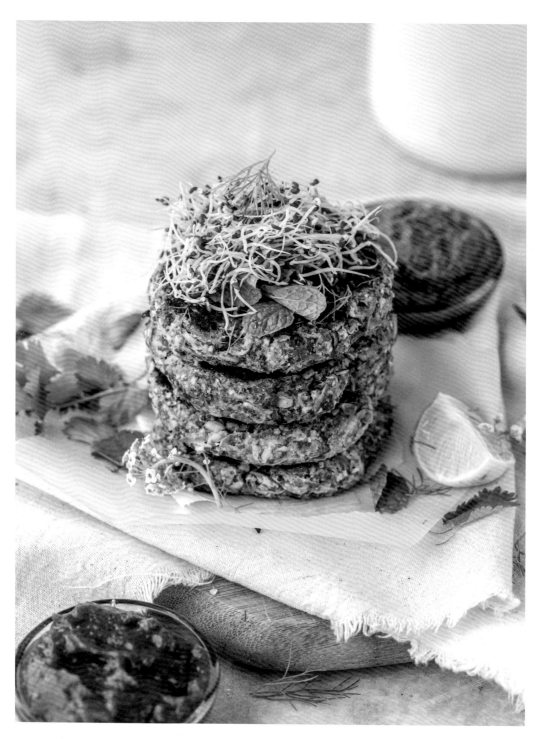

VEGETABLE TIKKI

BEST FOR

- ○ Morning Detox Drink
- ○ Breakfast
- ✓ Lunch
- ○ Mid-Meal
- ✓ Dinner
- ○ An Occasional Treat

These vegetable tikkis are made of only vegetables. We replaced potato with bottle guard to make the tikkis even lighter & more nutritious. They taste delicious paired with the chutneys.

INGREDIENTS
MAKES 7 TIKKIS

Vegetable tikki

- ¾ cup bottle guard, finely grated
- ½ cup cauliflower, chopped
- ⅛ cup green peas
- ⅛ cup carrot, chopped
- 1 ½ tablespoon flax seed, powdered*
- 1 tablespoon coriander, chopped
- ½ tablespoon mint leaves, chopped
- 1 teaspoon green chillies, finely chopped
- ½ teaspoon cumin seeds
- 1 teaspoon lemon juice
- ¼ teaspoon rock salt
- extra flax seed powder for rolling

*Flax seed powder is made by blending dry flax seeds in a blender.

Sweet Date Chutney (pg 91)

Green Chutney (pg 90)

METHOD

1. To prepare the tikkis, add all ingredients, except for salt and bottle guard, to your blender and blend till combined.

2. Take out this batter in a bowl.

3. Take the grated bottle gourd and squeeze out the water from it. Combine the squeezed bottle gourd with the batter.

4. Add salt to batter right before rolling tikkis.

5. Divide the mixture into 7 equal balls, and flatten each ball to form a thin tikki. Roll the tikkis in flax powder till evenly coated.

6. Heat a non-stick pan (griddle) and cook the tikkis on a medium flame. Press them using a spatula till they are fully cooked and turn golden brown from both sides. Do not use oil.

7. Serve hot with Sweet Date Chutney and Green Chutney.

Scan to watch the video

CHUTNEYS & DIPS

Here are three delicious chutneys to enhance the taste of your dishes.

- **Green Chutney** pairs well with all the Indian dishes - sabzi-roti, khichari, daliya and cheela.
- **Date Chutney** pairs well with the tikkis and cheela.
- **Coconut Chutney** can be served with cheela, upma and other south-indian dishes.

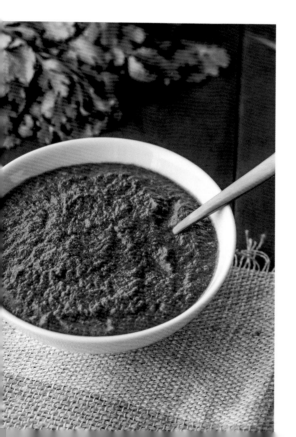

GREEN CHUTNEY

INGREDIENTS

- 1 cup coriander leaves
- ½ cup mint leaves
- ½ cup unripe mango, roughly chopped
- 1 teaspoon cumin seeds
- 1 teaspoon rock salt
- 1 small green chili

METHOD

1. Simply blend all ingredients together in a blender.
2. Store in the refrigerator for 2-3 days.

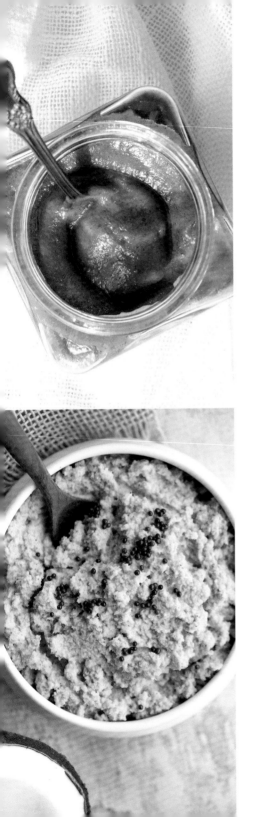

DATE CHUTNEY

INGREDIENTS

- ⅓ cup water
- 10 dates, seedless
- 2 teaspoons lemon juice
- 1 teaspoon cumin seeds
- 1 teaspoon rock salt
- 1 small green chili

METHOD

1. Simply blend all the ingredients together until smooth.
2. Store in the refrigerator for 2-3 days.

COCONUT CHUTNEY

INGREDIENTS

- 1 ½ cups chopped coconut
- ¼ cup chopped coriander
- ½ cup water
- 1 coin ginger, chopped
- 2 tablespoons roasted chickpeas (bhuna chana)
- 2 tablespoons soaked tamarind water
- ¼ green chilli, chopped
- 1 teaspoon rock salt
- 1 teaspoon black mustard seeds
- 6-8 curry leaves

METHOD

1. Simply blend all the ingredients (except the mustard seeds and curry leaves) in a blender.

2. Dry roast the mustard seeds and curry leaves and add them to the blended chutney from top.

3. Refrigerate the chutney for 20-30 minutes before use to get a refreshing taste.

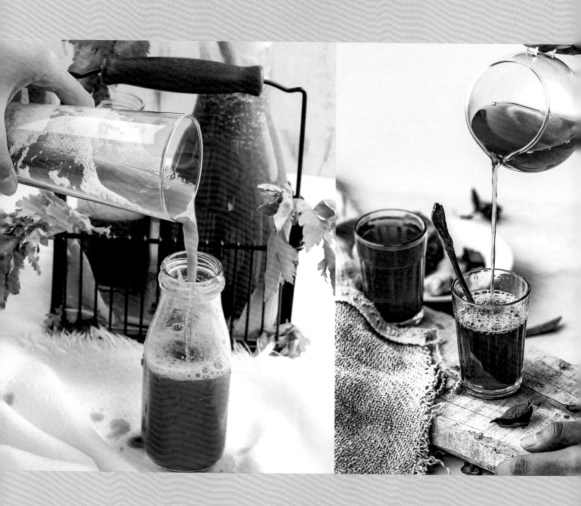

4th meal (optional)
MID-MEAL

About 2-3 hours after lunch, you might feel like snacking. At this time, we suggest that you stick to fresh juices. No namkeens, no biscuits, no chips. If fresh juices are not enough, you can have herbal tea, fresh coconut slices or a small piece of fruit.

MID - MEAL

MID-MEAL

During your mid-meal, you can repeat any of the juices from your morning detox juice, but make sure you take it out fresh again.

Juices are highly water-rich in nature. 70% of your diet should consist of water-rich foods. Juices cleanse your body by flushing out the waste in your intestines. While drinking juices, your body gets more of what it needs with less food. Introduce juicing as a culture in your life and you will see the benefits! Here are some juices you can drink in your mid-meal.

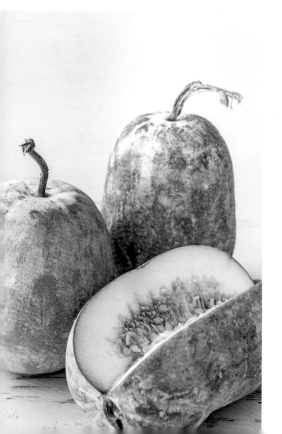

1st option (best option)

ASH GOURD JUICE

Ash gourd *(safed petha)* is one of the most detoxifying vegetables in Nature. When it enters our body, it starts to suck in all the toxins and when it leaves our body, it carries with it all the toxic waste. It is like a sponge in our digestive system. Many people tell that their stomach immediately gets cleared after drinking ash gourd juice.

Ash Gourd is easy to find at vegetable vendors. It belongs to the gourd family and is also called 'winter melon'. Don't worry, the taste of ash gourd juice is not bitter at all. In fact, it's quite bland, like water.

INGREDIENTS
Ash gourd *(safed petha)*

METHOD
1. Remove the peel of the ash gourd and take out all the seeds from inside.
2. Cut it into pieces and juice it. Drink about 400 ml (1 glass) of this juice every morning.

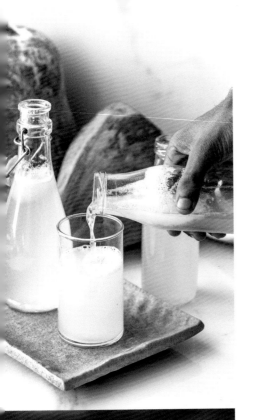

ASH COCO JUICE

If for some reason, you do not like the taste of ash gourd, or want to give it to children, you may mix the ash gourd juice with 50% coconut water.

INGREDIENTS

50% ash gourd juice
50% coconut water

METHOD

1. Mix the ash gourd juice with 50% coconut water.

2. Drink about 400 ml (1 glass) of this ash coco juice every morning.

MID - MEAL

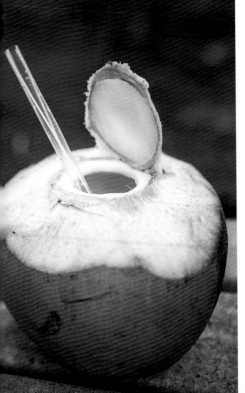

3rd best option

COCONUT WATER

Coconut is called "*Shree Phal*" in Sanskrit. It's the only fruit which is given the title *Shree* in front of it, because of it's healing properties. Coconut water is a natural laxative. Make sure you only use fresh coconut water, not the pre-packaged or bottled version. In case coconut water is not available in your country, you can drink the juice of any other fresh green vegetable - such as celery, cucumber, bottle gourd, spinach, etc.

INGREDIENTS

400 ml (about 1 glass) of coconut water

FRUIT / VEGETABLE JUICES

If you feel bored of drinking ash gourd juice and coconut water, you can give these fruit/vegetable juices a try. You can also make these if you decide to do a two or three day juice fast.

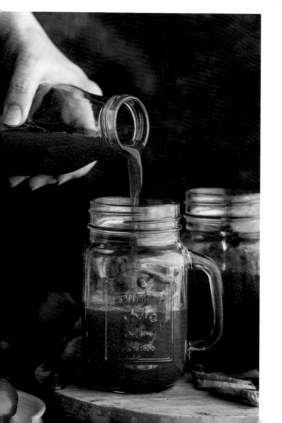

ABC JUICE
SERVES 2

INGREDIENTS

- 1 medium apple
- 2 medium beetroots
- 8 carrots
- 1 inch coin ginger

Substitution You can replace apples with pears.

METHOD

1. Simply juice all the ingredients together and serve.

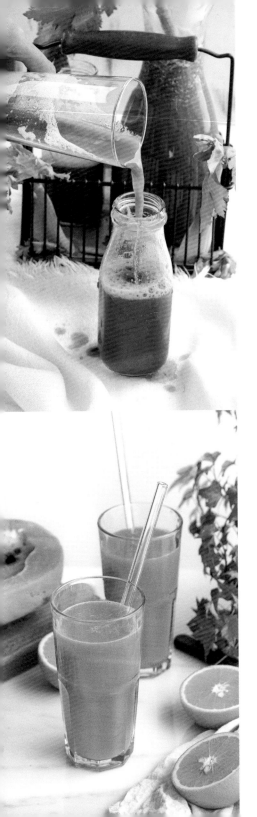

GLOWING GREEN JUICE
SERVES 2

INGREDIENTS

- 3 cups chopped cucumber or bottle gourd
- 1 cup roughly chopped spinach, tightly packed
- ¼ cup mint leaves, tightly packed
- 2 cups chopped apple
- 1 inch coin ginger
- 1 teaspoon lemon juice

METHOD

1. Simply juice all the ingredients together
2. Add the lemon juice from the top and serve.

Tip When juicing leafy greens like spinach and mint, alternate them with watery ingredients such as cucumber and apples. This helps your juicer to keep things moving.

CLEAN CARROT JUICE
SERVES 2

INGREDIENTS

- 2 cups chopped carrots
- 3 cups chopped papaya
- 2 oranges
- 1 inch coin ginger

Substitution You can replace oranges with kinnow.

METHOD

1. Simply juice all the ingredients together and serve.

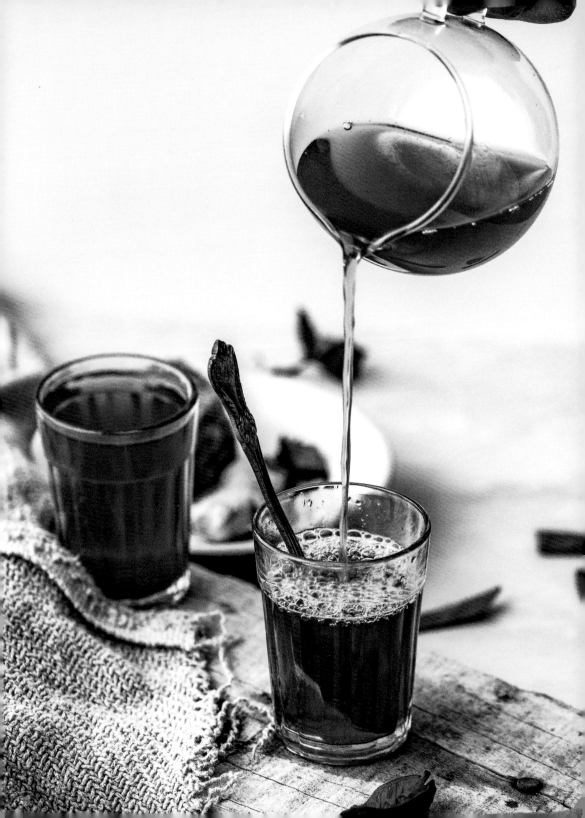

HERBAL TEA

BEST FOR

- ○ Morning Detox Drink
- ○ Breakfast
- ○ Lunch
- ✓ Mid-Meal
- ○ Dinner
- ○ An Occasional Treat

This herbal tea is a replacement for the traditional Indian tea made using milk and tea leaves. It helps get rid off tea addiction. It is made using a blend of herbs and natural flavors, without milk and tea leaves. You can use any fresh herb to make this tea - rosemary, curry leaves, tulsi, rose. We personally like lemongrass the most!

LEMONGRASS FLAVOR

INGREDIENTS
SERVES 2

- 2-3 inches of lemongrass stems, chopped
- Cinnamon sticks, 2 inches
- 6 green cardamom buds
- ½ inch coin ginger
- 2 cups water
- 1 teaspoon jaggery (optional)

Substitution Instead of lemongrass, you can use rosemary, curry leaves, tulsi or rose.

METHOD

1. Take a saucepan, add the water and bring it to a boil.

2. Crush the lemongrass steams, cinnamon sticks, cardamom buds & ginger in a mortar and pestle. Add to the water and cover the pan for 3 minutes, to let the flavors infuse.

3. Strain the tea through the strainer into cups.

4. If you like your tea sweetened, add jaggery from the top and serve.

Scan to watch
the video

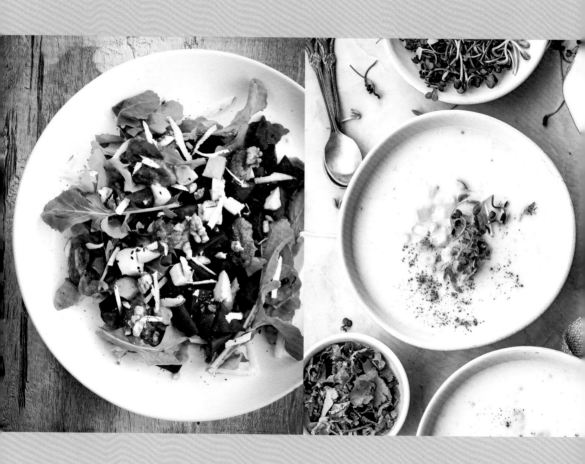

5th meal

DINNER

For dinner, have a light meal like a salad or soup. You can either have both (salad and soup) or only one (only salad or only soup), depending on your convenience. You may have fruits for dinner if you ate your salad meal for breakfast. You may have your grain meal for dinner if you ate your salad meal for lunch.

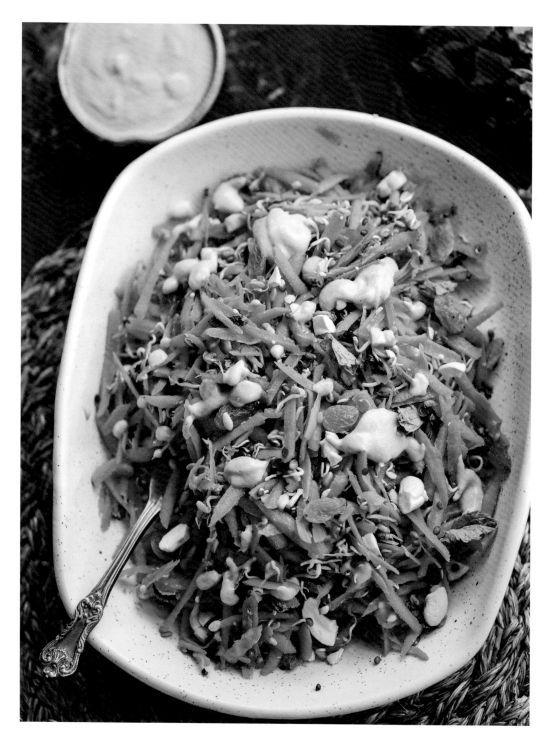

CARROT RAISIN SALAD

BEST FOR

○ Morning Detox Drink
○ Breakfast
✔ Lunch
○ Mid-Meal
✔ Dinner
○ An Occasional Treat

The ingredients are very simple & all easily available in any Indian Kitchen. The raisins, tahini and carrots combine together to create an absolutely yummy dish.

INGREDIENTS
SERVES 2 AS MAIN MEAL

- 3 cups shredded carrots
- 1 cup homegrown vegetable sprouts (such as alfalfa, clover, radish)
- 2 tablespoon finely chopped mint
- ¼ cup soaked cashews, chopped
- 3 tablespoons raisins (*kishmish*)

Tahini Dressing
- 1 cup white sesame seeds or 4 tablespoons homemade tahini
- ½ cup water
- 4 dates, seedless
- 2 tablespoons lemon juice
- 1 tablespoon powdered jaggery
- ¼ green chili
- ½ teaspoon rock salt

PRE-PREPARATION

Prepare vegetable sprouts as explained on pg 42.

METHOD

First, prepare the tahini.

1. To prepare tahini, add sesame seeds to a saucepan over medium heat and toast, stirring constantly until the seeds become fragrant and very lightly colored (not brown), 3 to 5 minutes. Careful, sesame seeds can burn quickly.

2. Once sesame seeds have been cooled, blend them until a paste forms, about 30 seconds. The tahini paste should be extra smooth, not gritty.

3. To prepare the dressing, place 4 tablespoons of this homemade tahini into a blender, along with water, dates, lemon juice, jaggery, chili and salt. Blend until smooth.

4. Place the carrots, sprouts, mint, cashews and raisins to a large mixing bowl. Mix well. Pour the tahini dressing on top and serve.

DINNER

Scan to watch the video

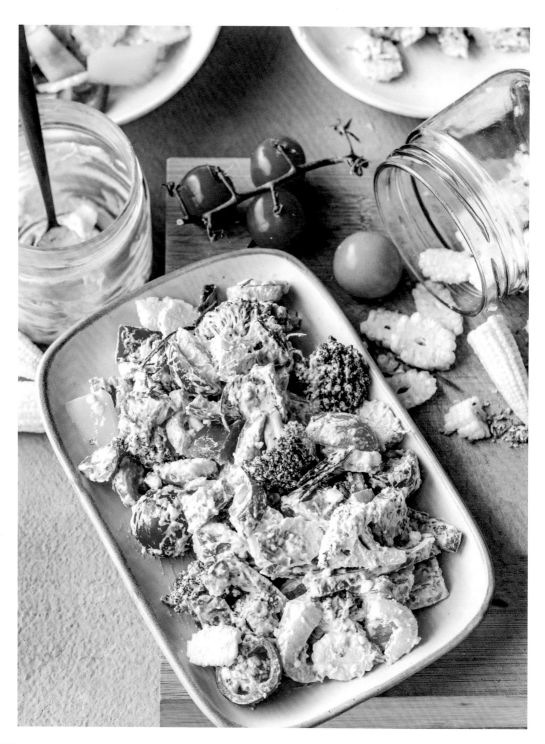

CHEESY SALAD

BEST FOR

○ Morning Detox Drink   ✓ Lunch   ✓ Dinner

○ Breakfast   ○ Mid-Meal   ○ An Occasional Treat

We don't need to use real cheese to get a cheesy flavor in your salad. Simply blend soaked cashews with some flavoring and it tastes even better than Parmesan!

INGREDIENTS

SERVES 2 (if served with a soup)

- ½ cup cashews. soaked
- ¼ cup coconut milk
- ½ small green chili
- 1 cup broccoli florets
- 1 cup thinly sliced baby corn
- 1 cup chopped red bell pepper
- 1 cup chopped yellow bell pepper
- 1 teaspoon rock salt
- 1 tablespoon dried oregano leaves

PRE-PREPARATION

- Soak cashews in water for 6 hours.
- Prepare coconut milk.

METHOD

1. Place the cashews, coconut milk and green chili into a blender and blend until smooth.

2. Steam the broccoli, baby corn and bell peppers for about 5 minutes. Bear in mind - bell peppers may get steamed faster and will need to be taken out sooner.

3. Pour the blended cashew mixture into a mixing bowl. Add the steamed vegetables, salt and oregano to the mixing bowl.

4. Mix well and serve.

DINNER

Scan to watch
the video

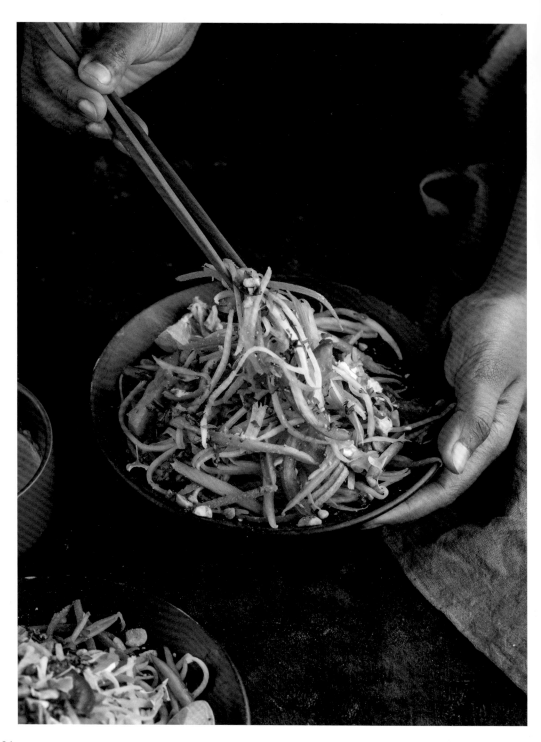

THAI PAPAYA SALAD

BEST FOR

○ Morning Detox Drink   ☑ Lunch   ☑ Dinner
○ Breakfast   ○ Mid-Meal   ○ An Occasional Treat

Papaya salad gets its inspiration from Thai Cuisine. This is a cleaner version of the dish, made using only fresh, wholesome ingredients. It is crunchy and amazingly delicious.

INGREDIENTS
SERVES 2-3

- ½ small unripe green papaya
- 1 large mango
- 1 medium carrot
- 2 medium tomatoes
- ½ cup fresh coriander

Peanut Dressing (makes ⅓ cup)

- 2 tablespoons soaked peanuts
- 1 tablespoon lemon juice
- ⅛ small green chili
- ½ teaspoon rock salt
- 1 tablespoon jaggery
- 2 tablespoons water

Topping

- 1 tablespoon roasted peanuts, chopped

Substitution When mango is not in season, use a soft pear.

PRE-PREPARATION

Soak raw peanuts in water for about 3 hours.

METHOD

1. Peel the skin of the papaya.
2. Cut the papaya and carrot into thin long strips. You can use a julienne peeler to do this.
3. Also cut the mango and tomatoes into thin long strips, using a knife.
4. Place the papaya, carrot, mango, tomatoes and coriander in a large bowl and mix well.
5. To prepare the dressing, place all the dressing ingredients into a blender and blend until smooth.
6. Combine the dressing with the salad and mix well.
7. Top with chopped peanuts for an extra crunch.

Tip The papaya used is unripe green papaya, which is green on the outside and a pale yellowish color on the inside.

DINNER

Scan to watch the video

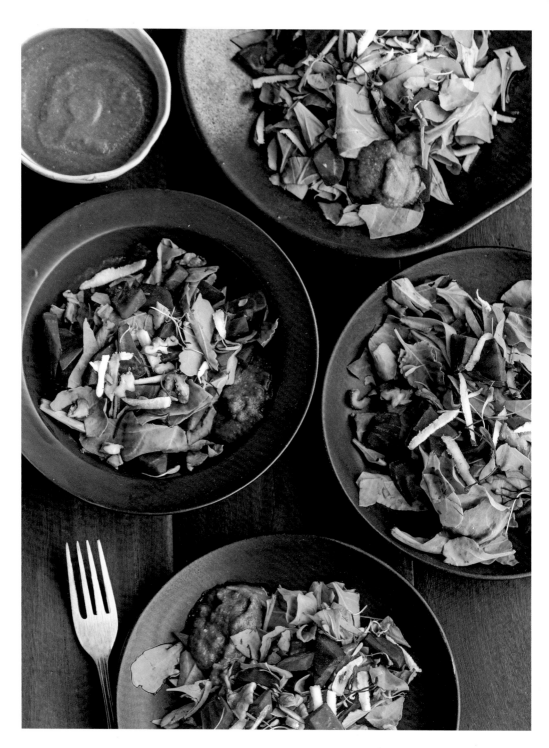

BEET ROCKET SALAD

BEST FOR

- ◯ Morning Detox Drink
- ◯ Breakfast
- ✅ Lunch
- ◯ Mid-Meal
- ✅ Dinner
- ◯ An Occasional Treat

This is a quick and simple salad that tastes wonderfully gourmet. Rocket leaves have a spicy, mustard-like flavor that is balanced out by the dates and beetroot.

INGREDIENTS
SERVES 2

- 2 small beetroot, peeled
- 2 cups chopped spinach leaves
- 1 cup chopped rocket leaves
- 6 walnuts, soaked and crushed
- ¼ cup grated coconut
- ½ avocado, chopped (optional)

Middle Eastern Dressing

- ½ cup chopped cucumber
- 4 dates, seedless
- ¼ cup coriander
- 1½ tablespoon lemon juice
- ¼ teaspoon cumin powder

Substitution In case rocket leaves are not available, replace them with spinach leaves.

METHOD

1. Chop the beetroot and steam it until soft.

2. Place the steamed beetroot into a large mixing bowl, along with the spinach, rocket, coconut, walnuts and avocado (optional).

3. To prepare the Middle Eastern Dressing, place all the dressing ingredients into a blender and blend until smooth.

4. Pour the dressing over the salad, toss well and serve.

Tip Add vegetable sprouts to the salad for maximum nutrition (See page 42).

DINNER

Scan to watch
the video

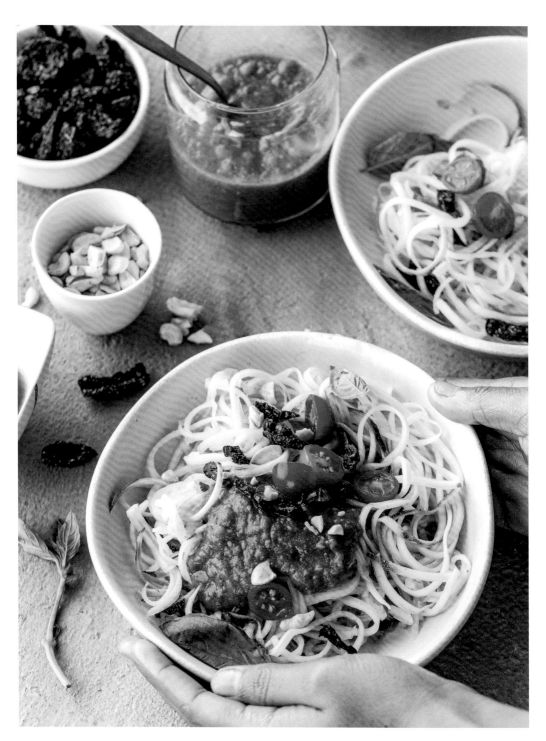

ZUCCHINI SPAGHETTI

BEST FOR

- ◯ Morning Detox Drink
- ◯ Breakfast
- ✅ Lunch
- ◯ Mid-Meal
- ✅ Dinner
- ◯ An Occasional Treat

One of my favorite things to create in the kitchen are zucchini noodles. Using raw vegetables in place of conventional cooked pasta is a great way to eat more vegetables. Since this dish is raw, it loaded with nutrients and living enzymes. Serve with a fresh green salad for a satisfying meal that almost anyone will love.

INGREDIENTS
SERVES 3 (if served with a soup)

Spaghetti Sauce

- 1½ cup cherry tomatoes
- 6 dates, seedless
- 1½ tablespoon oregano
- 3 tablespoons fresh basil leaves or 1 teaspoon dry basil
- 1½ tablespoon lemon juice
- 2 teaspoons rock salt

Zucchini Noodles

- 3 medium zucchinis

Topping

- 1 tablespoon crushed cashews
- 1 tablespoon thinly sliced sun-dried tomatoes
- 8 cherry tomatoes, cut into halves
- ¼ cup basil leaves

METHOD

1. To make the spaghetti sauce, place all the sauce ingredients in a blender and blend until well combined.

2. To make the zucchini noodles, use a vegetable spiraliser (See page 41) and make spaghetti-style noodles.

3. Right before serving, stir the spaghetti sauce through the zucchini noodles. Do not combine the sauce and zucchini too much in advance or the zucchini will release water.

4. Top with cashews, sun-dried tomatoes, cherry tomatoes and basil. Serve.

Scan to watch
the video

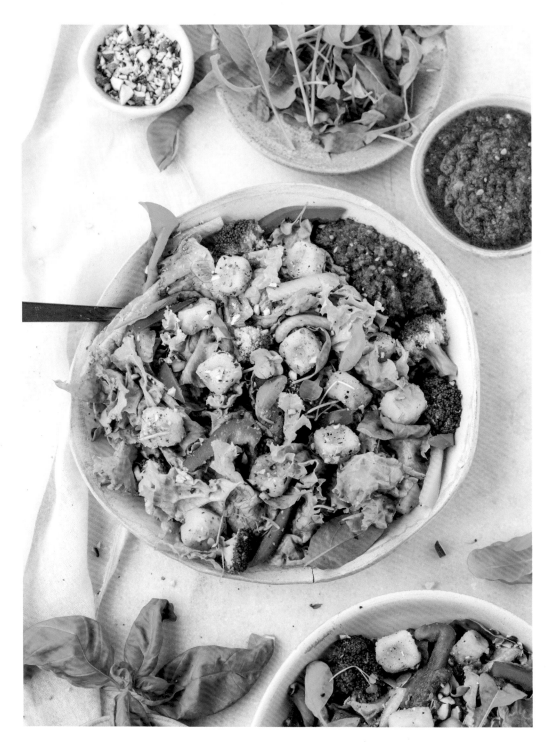

SWEET POTATO SALAD

BEST FOR

○ Morning Detox Drink ✓ Lunch ✓ Dinner
○ Breakfast ○ Mid-Meal ○ An Occasional Treat

INGREDIENTS

SERVES 2-3

- 1 medium sweet potato, steamed
- 2 cups lettuce leaves, torn into pieces
- 1½ cup broccoli, cut into florets
- ¼ small red bell pepper,
  thinly sliced & then cut half
- ¼ small yellow bell pepper,
  thinly sliced and then cut half
- 1 tablespoon dry rosemary

For marinating sweet potato

- 1 tablespoon lemon juice
- ¼ teaspoon black pepper
- ½ teaspoon salt

Tomato Salsa Dressing

- 2 cups frozen tomatoes,
  peeled & seedless
- ¼ cup coriander
- 1 tablespoon chopped red bell pepper
- ½ teaspoon roasted cumin powder
- ½ teaspoon lemon juice
- ½ green chilli, chopped
- ½ teaspoon rock salt
- ⅛ teaspoon black pepper

Topping

- 2 tablespoons dry roasted almonds,
  chopped finely

PRE-PREPARATION

Freeze the tomatoes for about 40-50
minutes to get a refreshing salsa flavour.

METHOD

For the salad

1. Peel the steamed sweet potato and
   mash it using a fork.

2. Add rosemary to the mashed potatoes
   and mix well. Using your hand, shape
   the mashed potatoes into small cubes.

3. Mix all the marination ingredients
   together and dip the sweet potato
   cubes in it till coated from all sides.

4. Meanwhile, dip the broccoli in water
   heated on a medium flame for 10 mins.

5. Combine the lettuce, bell peppers,
   steamed broccoli and marinated sweet
   potatoes in a mixing bowl.

For the dressing

6. Blend all the dressing ingredients in the
   blender. Don't blend it too much. Keep
   it a little chunky. Refrigerate the dressing
   for a refreshing taste before use.

7. Pour the dressing on top of the salad.
   Top with toasted almonds & enjoy!

DINNER

Scan to watch
the video

113

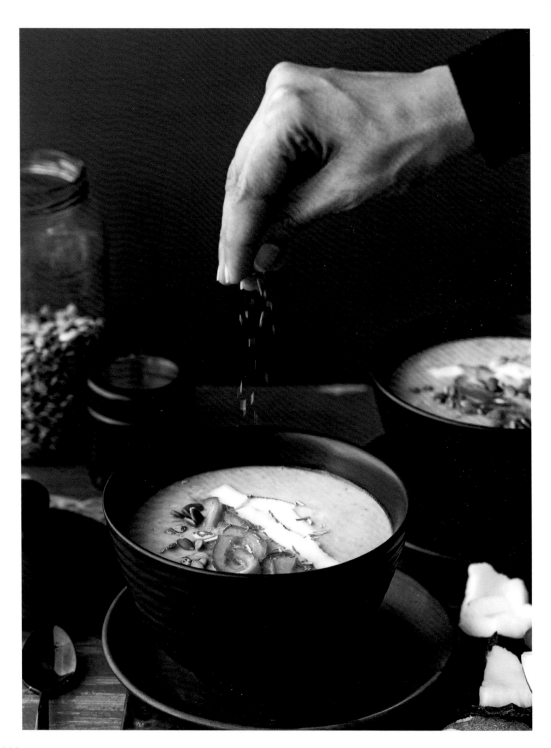

PUMPKIN SOUP

BEST FOR

○ Morning Detox Drink ✓ Lunch ✓ Dinner
○ Breakfast ○ Mid-Meal ○ An Occasional Treat

This pumpkin soup ticks all the boxes! Its rich, creamy and ultimately satisfying. The rosemary & thyme combine to create a unique flavor, which you may have never experienced before.

DINNER

INGREDIENTS
SERVES 2, MAKES 1200 ml

Soup Base

- ½ kg red pumpkin, with peel
- 3 cups coconut milk
- 2 tablespoons fresh thyme or 2 teaspoons dry thyme
- 1 stem fresh rosemary or ½ teaspoon dry rosemary
- 2 teaspoons rock salt
- ½ small green chili, chopped

Toppings

- 2 tablespoons pumpkin seeds
- ½ red bell pepper, cut into strips
- ¼ small coconut, cut into strips

PRE-PREPARATION

Prepare coconut milk.

METHOD

1. Chop the pumpkin into chunks. Do not take the peel off. Add it to a steamer and let it steam for about 20 minutes, until soft.

2. Once the pumpkin has cooled, place it in a blender, along with the coconut milk, thyme, rosemary, salt and chili. Blend until smooth.

3. Pour the soup into bowls, add the toppings from above and serve.

Tip Do not re-heat the soup because we should never cook coconut or coconut milk on the stove.

Tip Make sure you add rosemary and thyme to this soup, since they carry all the flavor. In case fresh is not available, use their dried versions.

Scan to watch
the video

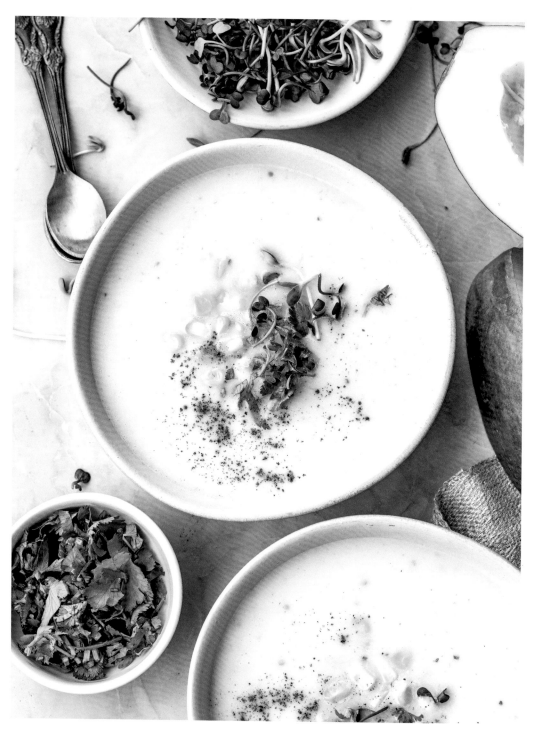

PAPAYA CORN SOUP

BEST FOR

○ Morning Detox Drink
○ Breakfast

✔ Lunch
○ Mid-Meal

✔ Dinner
○ An Occasional Treat

INGREDIENTS
SERVES 2, MAKES 1400 ml

Soup Base
- 3 cups peeled & chopped green papaya (approximately 1 small green papaya)
- ½ small green chili, chopped
- 2 teaspoons coriander seeds
- 1 teaspoon chopped ginger
- 1½ tablespoons chopped lemongrass stalks
- 2 ¼ cups water
- 1½ tablespoon lemon juice
- 2 teaspoons rock salt
- 1 cup coconut milk

Topping
- ¼ cup corn, boiled
- ¼ cup chopped coriander

PRE-PREPARATION
Prepare coconut milk.

METHOD

1. Steam the papaya until it is soft.

2. Meanwhile, take a shallow pan and dry roast the green chili, coriander seeds, ginger and lemongrass together. Add ¼ cup water and let them cook together for 2-3 minutes, till the flavors are soaked in.

3. Place this spice mixture in a blender along with the steamed papaya, 2 cups water, lemon juice and salt. Blend until absolutely smooth.

4. Right before serving, add coconut milk to the soup. Stir well.

5. Top with corn and coriander and serve (Do not re-heat before serving).

Tip The papaya used is not the soft, ripe and orangey one, but the unripened green papaya, which is firm, green on the outside and white on the inside.

DINNER

Scan to watch
the video

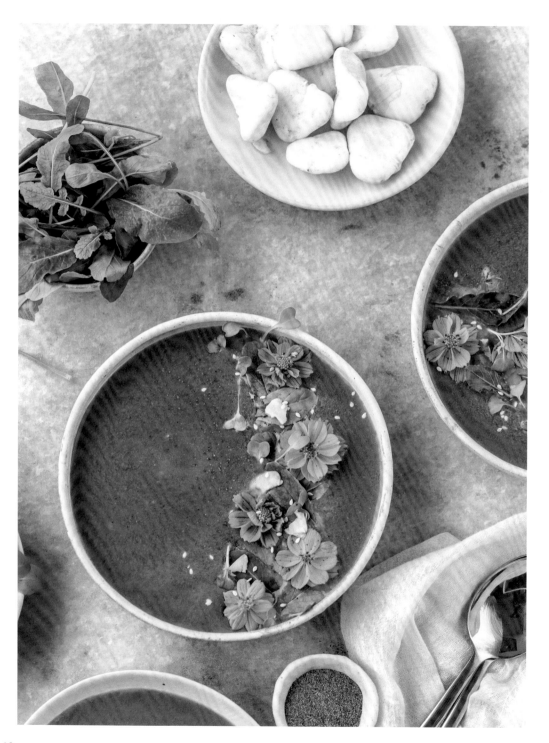

SPINACH SINGHARA SOUP

BEST FOR

- ◯ Morning Detox Drink
- ◯ Breakfast
- ✅ Lunch
- ◯ Mid-Meal
- ✅ Dinner
- ◯ An Occasional Treat

This soup is a staple in my home. It's hearty and comforting. The coconut milk gives it a subtle sweetness and also helps to thicken it.

INGREDIENTS
SERVES 2, MAKES 1400 ml

Soup Base

- ½ kg spinach
- 3 cups water
- ¾ cup *singhara* (water chestnuts) peeled and thinly sliced
- 2½ teaspoons rock salt
- ½ teaspoon black pepper
- ½ cup coconut milk

Garnish

- microgreens (optional)
- mary gold petals (optional)

Substitution In case *singhara* is not available, use potato.

PRE-PREPARATION

Prepare coconut milk.

METHOD

1. Place the spinach and water in a pan. Heat on a low flame till the spinach is soft (about 15 minutes).

2. Puree this mixture using a hand blender, till smooth.

3. Pour this blended mixture through a sieve to get any stalks out.

4. Keep the blended mixture back on the stove, on a low flame. Add the thinly sliced *singhara* and keep on a low flame for about 3 minutes.

5. Turn off the heat and add salt and pepper.

6. Right before serving, add the coconut milk to your soup and stir well.

7. Garnish with microgreens (optional) and serve. Do not re-heat the soup after adding coconut mllk.

DINNER

119

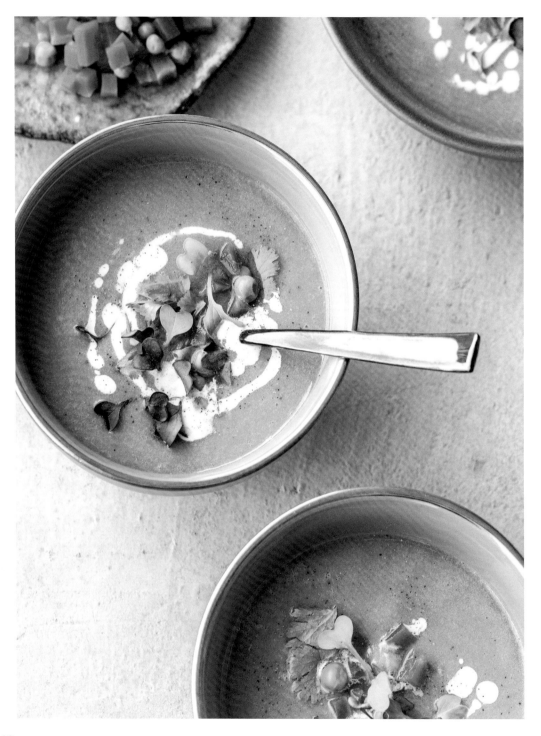

PEA CARROT SOUP

BEST FOR

- ○ Morning Detox Drink
- ○ Breakfast
- ☑ Lunch
- ○ Mid-Meal
- ☑ Dinner
- ○ An Occasional Treat

INGREDIENTS

SERVES 2, MAKES 900 ml

Soup Base

- 1 cup fresh peas
- 1 cup chopped carrot
- ½ cup chopped potatoes
- 2 small bay leaves
- ½ inch coin of ginger, chopped
- 3 cups of water
- 2 teaspoons lemon juice
- 2 teaspoons rock salt

Topping

- ½ cup fresh peas
- ½ cup chopped carrots, diced
- ¼ cup chopped coriander

METHOD

Soup Base

1. Place the peas, carrots, potatoes, bay leaves, ginger, and water into a pan, cover and cook on a low flame for about 15 minutes, until all vegetables are soft.

2. Remove bay leaves from the pan.

3. Using a hand blender, puree the vegetables till smooth.

4. Add lemon juice and salt from the top.

Topping

1. Steam/boil the peas and carrots until soft.

2. Add the boiled peas, carrots and coriander into the soup base. Stir well and serve warm.

Note Use only fresh peas (not frozen peas) and red winter carrots to make this soup.

DINNER

Scan to watch
the video

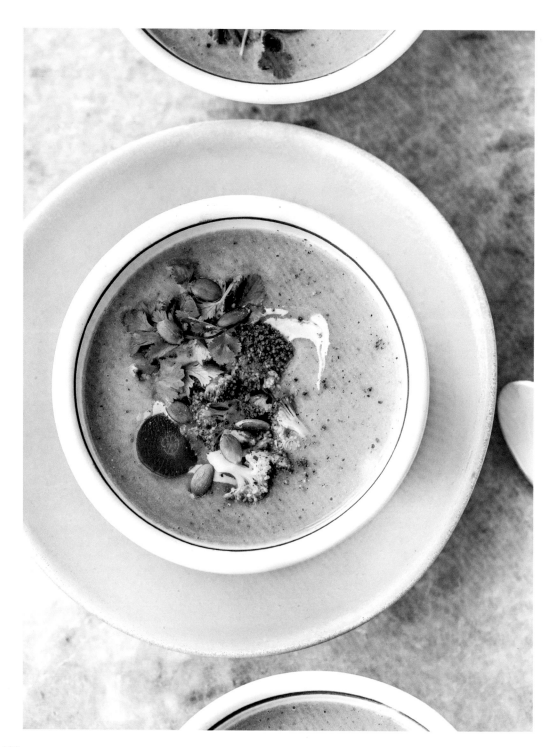

BROCCOLI POTATO SOUP

BEST FOR

○ Morning Detox Drink   ✅ Lunch   ✅ Dinner
○ Breakfast   ○ Mid-Meal   ○ An Occasional Treat

This rustic broccoli & potato soup is the perfect winter warmer. It is so easy to make with just a few simple ingredients but it's full of flavour and hearty goodness.

INGREDIENTS
SERVES 2-3, MAKES 1½ litres

Soup Base
- 2½ cups fresh broccoli, roughly cut
- 1½ cups potatoes, roughly cut
- 3 cups water
- 1½ teaspoons rock salt
- 1 inch fresh ginger, grated
- ¼ teaspoon black pepper powder
- 1 cup coconut milk

Topping
- 1 cup fresh broccoli, roughly cut
- ½ carrot, cut into circles
- ¼ cup fresh coriander, chopped
- 1 tablespoon pumpkin seeds

PRE-PREPARATION
Prepare coconut milk.

METHOD

Soup Base

1. Heat a saucepan over medium heat. Add the broccoli, potato and water. Cover the pot and let the vegetables cook for 20 minutes, or until the potatoes are fork tender.

2. Add the ginger to the saucepan and let it cook with the vegetables for another 3-4 minutes.

3. Remove the pot from the stove and use an immersion blender to puree the vegetables.

4. Add the salt and pepper and mix well.

5. Right before serving, add the coconut milk.

Topping

6. Steam the broccoli and carrot until soft. Add to your soup, along with coriander and pumpkin seeds. Serve the soup warm.

DINNER

Scan to watch
the video

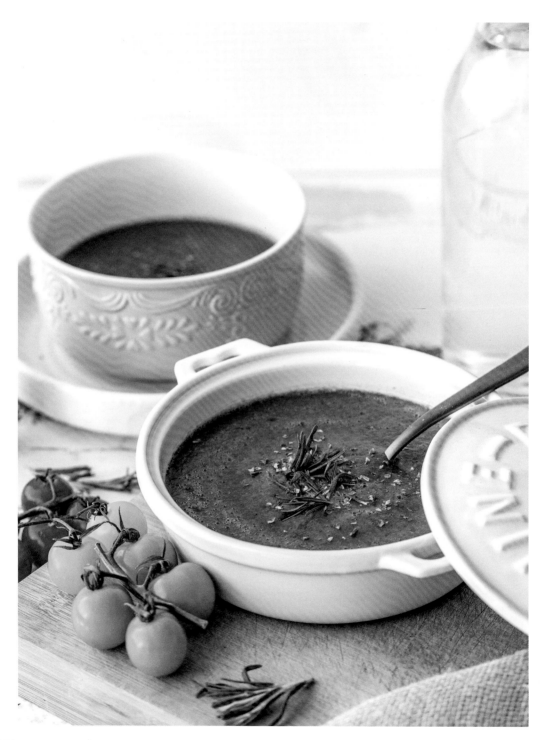

TOMATO SOUP

BEST FOR

○ Morning Detox Drink ✓ Lunch ✓ Dinner
○ Breakfast ○ Mid-Meal ○ An Occasional Treat

In Satvic cuisine, we do not cook tomatoes. We always add them in the end, because tomatoes are rich in Vitamin C, which is a very delicate vitamin and gets destroyed easily when heated. Therefore, in this soup, we only blanch the tomatoes, to preserve their nutrition.

INGREDIENTS

SERVES 1-2. MAKES 700 ml

- 8 medium tomatoes
- ¼ cup chopped bottle gourd
- ¼ cup chopped carrot
- ¼ cup chopped potato
- ¼ cup chopped red bell pepper
- 1½ cups water
- ½ teaspoon dry rosemary
- ¾ teaspoon rock salt
- ¼ teaspoon black pepper powder
- ½ teaspoon dry oregano

METHOD

1. Dip the tomatoes in hot water for 15 minutes. Cover with a plate. After 15 minutes, peel off their skin and take out the seedy part from inside.

2. Heat a saucepan over medium heat. Add the bottle gourd, carrot, potato, bell pepper and 1½ cups of water. Cover the pot and let the vegetables cook for 15 minutes.

3. Add these vegetables and water to a blender, along with the peeled and de-seeded tomatoes and rosemary. Blend until smooth.

4. Mix in the salt, pepper and oregano. Serve.

DINNER

Scan to watch
the video

125

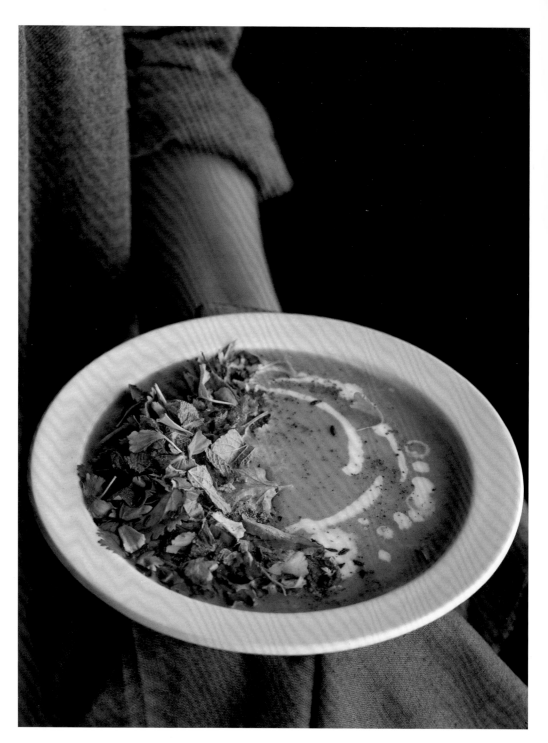

126

CARROT CUMIN SOUP

BEST FOR

○ Morning Detox Drink
○ Breakfast

☑ Lunch
○ Mid-Meal

☑ Dinner
○ An Occasional Treat

INGREDIENTS

SERVES 2, MAKES 1 litre

Soup Base

- 1 teaspoon cumin seeds
- 1 inch coin of ginger, chopped
- ½ teaspoon coriander powder
- 2 cups chopped carrots
- 1 cup cauliflower florets
- 3 cups water
- 1 bay leaf
- 1 cups coconut milk
- 2 teaspoons rock salt
- ½ teaspoon black pepper

Topping

- 2 tablespoons chopped coriander
- 2 tablespoons chopped mint

PRE-PREPARATION

Prepare coconut milk.

METHOD

1. Heat a saucepan over medium heat. Add cumin seeds, ginger and coriander powder. Stir well and cook for one minute, till the spices become fragrant.

2. Add diced carrot & cauliflower to the saucepan & cook for 5 mins while stirring occasionally.

3. Pour in the water and add the bay leaf. Bring to a boil. Partially cover the pot with a lid, reduce the heat to medium and simmer for 20 minutes.

4. Blend the ingredients in the saucepan using a hand-blender.

5. Add salt and pepper. Stir well.

6. Right before serving, add coconut milk and stir.

7. Garnish with coriander and mint. Serve warm.

DINNER

Scan to watch
the video

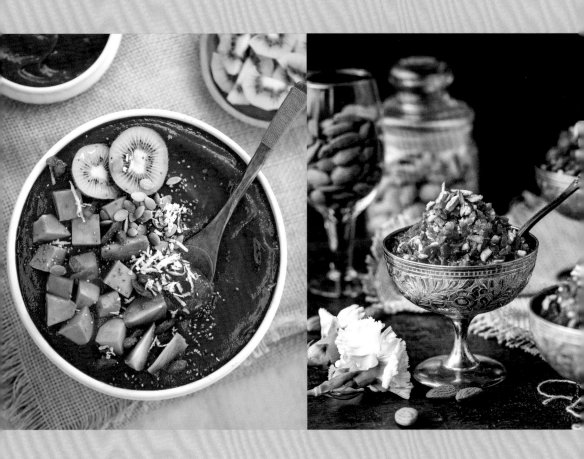

RECIPES FOR
SPECIAL OCCASIONS

The upcoming pages include exotic and delicious recipes that you can make at Satvic parties and festivals to inspire your friends and family to join you in this beautiful way of living and eating in sync with Mother Nature.

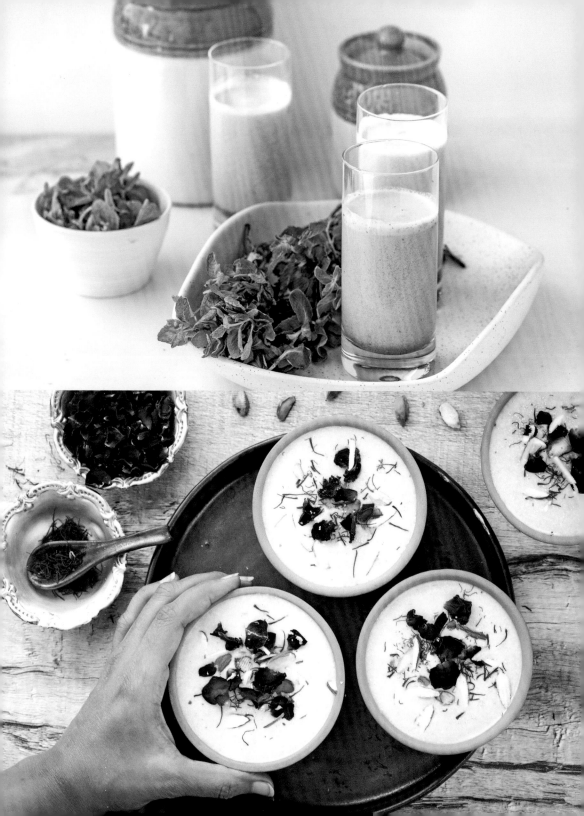

COCONUT CHAAS

INGREDIENTS
SERVES 2, MAKES 750 ml

Scan to watch
the video

- 2 cups coconut milk
- 1 cup water
- ¼ cup mint leaves
- 2 ½ tablespoon lemon juice
- 1 teaspoon rock salt
- 1 teaspoon roasted cumin powder (bhuna jeera powder)

METHOD

1. Place everything except the roasted cumin powder into a blender and blend until smooth.

2. And the roasted cumin powder from the top. Stir well. Let it cool in the refrigerator for a while and serve.

THANDAI

INGREDIENTS
SERVES 3, MAKES 600 ml

Scan to watch
the video

- 8 almonds, soaked in water & drained
- 1 tablespoon fennel, soaked in water for 1 hour & drained
- 1 tablespoon poppy seeds, soaked in water for 1 hour & drained
- 1½ cups coconut milk
- ½ cup water
- 4 dates, seedless
- 1 teaspoon powdered jaggery
- ⅛ teaspoon rock salt
- ⅛ teaspoon black pepper
  Garnishing
- chopped pistachio, saffron & dried rose petals

METHOD

1. Place everything except coconut milk into a blender and blend until smooth.
2. Add coconut milk and blend again.
3. Let the drink cool in the refrigerator for a while. Garnish & serve.

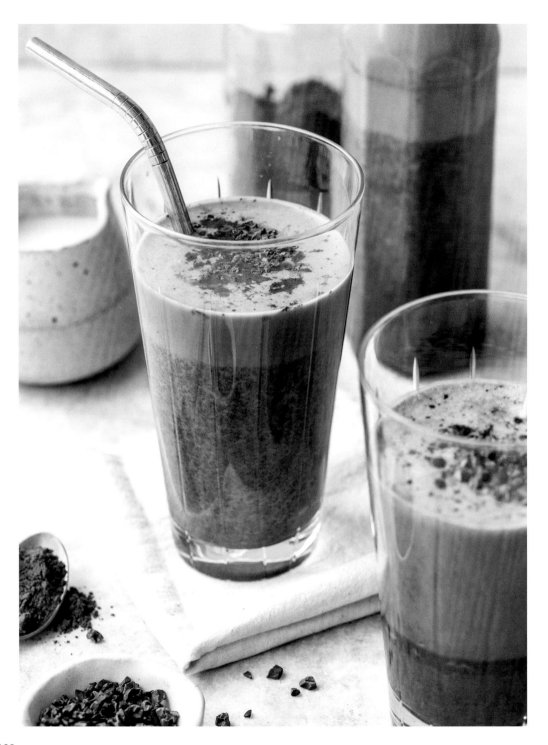

NO-COFFEE COLD-COFFEE

BEST FOR

○ Morning Detox Drink   ○ Lunch   ○ Dinner

○ Breakfast   ○ Mid-Meal   ☑ An Occasional Treat

We feel tired, gulp down a cup of coffee & become suddenly awake, but we have not suddenly become well rested & energetic. Coffee is a very strong stimulant. It brings us up and then suddenly dumps us down. Overtime, every cup of coffee makes our body weaker & weaker.

Here we have an unexpected substitute for coffee! It not just tastes like coffee, but even smells exactly like it. Even people from far away want to come and try it! Tell your friends that there's no dairy, sugar or coffee powder in their mugs, and they'll be busy guessing what's inside.

Bear in mind - you should have this coffee only occasionally (not more than once a week). Although it matches coffee perfectly in taste and smell, it is still not a healing food.

INGREDIENTS

Coffee Powder

• 100 gm chickpeas (*chole*)

Cold Coffee

SERVES 1

• 1 cup coconut milk keep in freezer for 3 hours

• 3 dates, seedless

• 1 teaspoon coffee powder

METHOD

Method for making coffee powder

1. Take a pan & roast the chickpeas on a medium flame. Continuously stir for at least 20 minutes, until the chickpeas become **dark brown** all across. Keep stirring continuously, otherwise they may burn. Make sure they are dark chocolatey brown, otherwise you will not get the coffee flavour.

2. Let the chickpeas cool. Then, place them in a mixer and grind them till they become a powder.

3. Then sieve them and store the sieved powder in an air tight container in the fridge.

Method for making cold coffee

4. Place the coconut milk, dates & coffee powder in a blender & blend until smooth.

5. Pour in glasses and serve.

OCCASIONAL

Scan to watch
the video

133

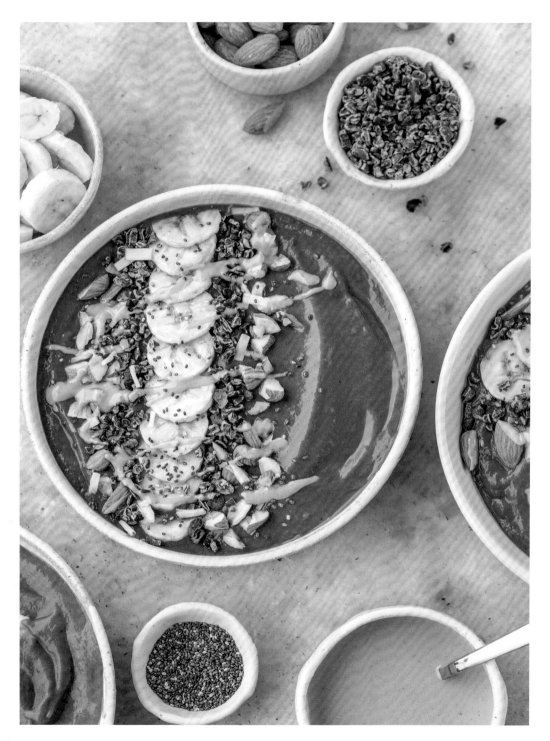

CHOCOLATE SMOOTHIE BOWL

BEST FOR

○ Morning Detox Drink
○ Breakfast

○ Lunch
○ Mid-Meal

○ Dinner
✔ An Occasional Breakfast

Blend cacao with some bananas, coconut milk and dates and you'll have a delicious ice-cream like smoothie bowl ready. This is undoubtedly, one of my favourite recipes in the book!

INGREDIENTS
SERVES 2

- 4 frozen bananas
- ½ cup coconut milk
- 2 tablespoons cacao powder
- 4 dates, seedless
- Pinch rock salt
- Pinch cinnamon powder
- 1 tablespoon peanut butter (optional)
- Pinch vanilla powder (optional)

Topping
- any seasonal fruits & nuts

PRE-PREPARATION

- Take the bananas, peel, slice and put in the freezer for about 6 hours.

METHOD

1. Place all the smoothie ingredients into a blender and blend until smooth.

2. Pour into bowls and top with fresh seasonal fruits and nuts of your choice.

* **Tip** Nuts and seeds are great to add texture to your bowl, but eat them minimally as they are water-poor in nature. Focus on fresh, water-rich fruits for your topping.

Scan to watch
the video

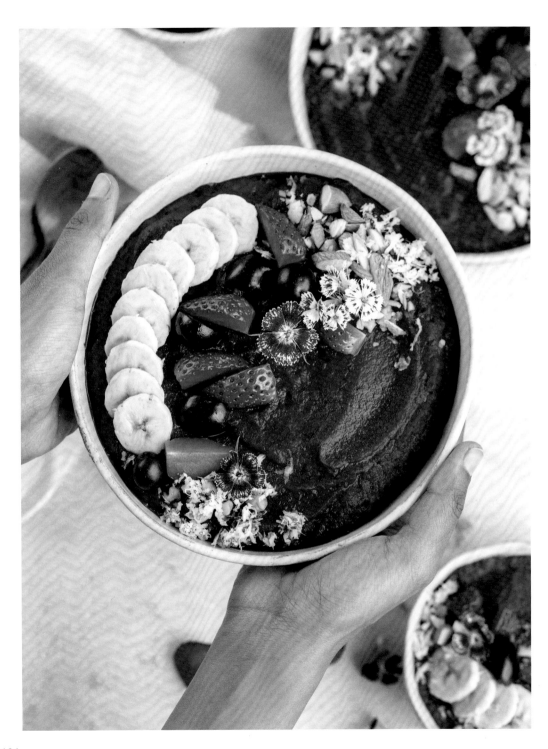

BLUSH SMOOTHIE BOWL

BEST FOR

○ Morning Detox Drink
○ Breakfast

○ Lunch
○ Mid-Meal

○ Dinner
✓ An Occasional Breakfast

I love the bright pink colour of this bowl. Get your kids involved in making it and they'll love watching the fruits blend together to create a yummy vibrant breakfast!

INGREDIENTS
SERVES 2

- 2 frozen bananas
- 3 chopped soft pears*
- ½ cup chopped beetroot

Topping
- any seasonal fruits & nuts

Substitution
In case pear is not available, use soft apples.

PRE-PREPARATION

Take the bananas, peel, slice and put in the freezer for about 6 hours.

METHOD

1. Place the pears, beetroot and frozen bananas in a blender and blend until smooth.

2. Pour into bowls and top with fresh seasonal fruits and nuts of your choice.

   Tip Nuts and seeds are great to add texture to your bowl, but eat them minimally as they are water-poor in nature. Focus on fresh, water-rich fruits for your topping.

   Tip Make sure you use the soft variety of pears. They should sink in a little when pressed with your thumb.

Scan to watch
the video

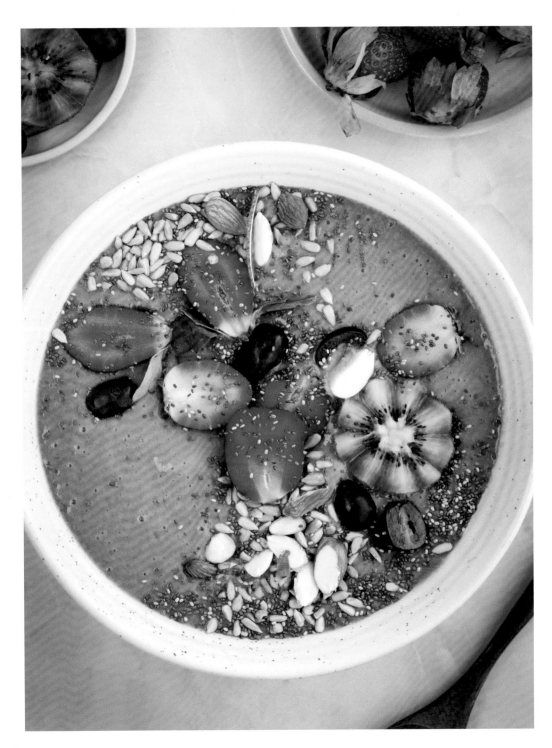

138

SPINACH SMOOTHIE BOWL

BEST FOR

○ Morning Detox Drink   ○ Lunch   ○ Dinner

○ Breakfast   ○ Mid-Meal   ✅ An Occasional Breakfast

This smoothie bowl is delicious and simple, requiring just 10 minutes to make. It is raw and only made using fruits and vegetables.

INGREDIENTS
SERVES 2

- 4 frozen bananas
- ¾ cup shredded coconut
- 2 cups of spinach
- 4 dates, seedless
- ½ teaspoon cinnamon powder
- 2 teaspoons lemon juice

Topping
- any seasonal fruits & nuts

PRE-PREPARATION

Take the bananas, peel, slice and put in the freezer for about 6 hours.

METHOD

1. Place the shredded coconut, spinach, dates, cinnamon, lemon juice and frozen bananas in a blender and blend until smooth.

2. Pour into bowls and top with fresh seasonal fruits and nuts of your choice.

- **Tip** Nuts and seeds are great to add texture to your bowl, but eat them minimally as they are water-poor in nature. Focus on fresh, water-rich fruits for your topping.

Scan to watch the video

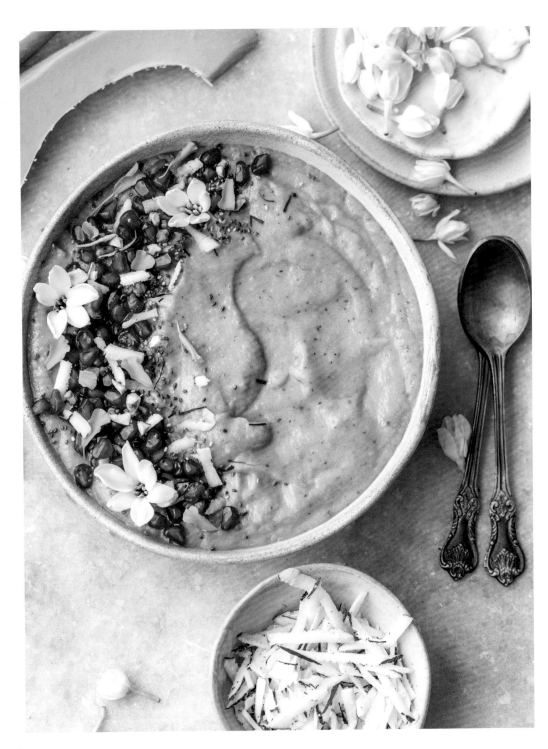

MARIGOLD SMOOTHIE BOWL

BEST FOR

○ Morning Detox Drink
○ Breakfast

○ Lunch
○ Mid-Meal

○ Dinner
◉ An Occasional Breakfast

Who thought saffron could go well in a smoothie bowl? Well, pair with some papaya and you'll have a delicious & unique smoothie base.

INGREDIENTS
SERVES 1

- 1½ cup frozen papaya
- 1 frozen banana
- 3 dates, seedless
- 6 strands saffron
- ¼ cup coconut milk

Topping
- any seasonal fruits & nuts

PRE-PREPARATION

Take papaya and banana. Peel, slice and put them in the freezer for about 6 hours.

METHOD

1. Place the frozen papaya, banana, dates, saffron and coconut milk in a blender and blend until smooth.

2. Pour this smoothie base into bowls, and top with any fresh seasonal fruits and nuts.

- **Tip** Nuts and seeds are great to add texture to your bowl, but eat them minimally as they are water-poor in nature. Focus on fresh, water-rich fruits for your topping.

Scan to watch the video

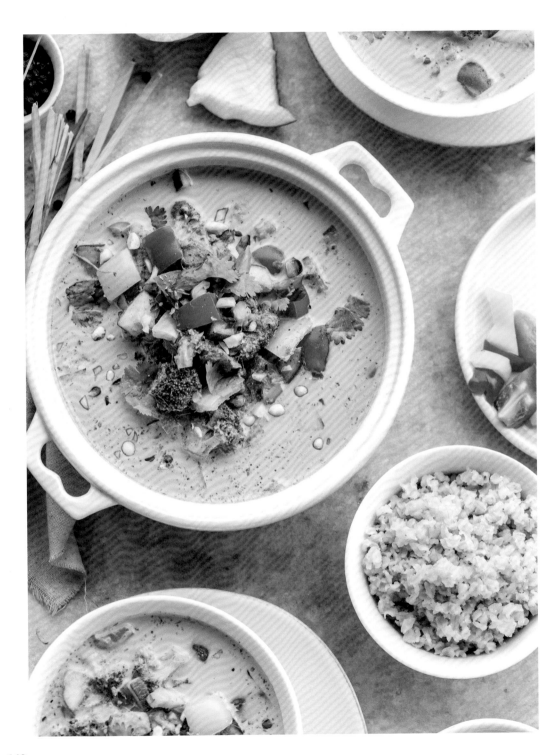

THAI CURRY WITH BROWN RICE

BEST FOR

- ○ Morning Detox Drink
- ○ Breakfast
- ○ Lunch
- ○ Mid-Meal
- ○ Dinner
- ◉ An Occasional Lunch

INGREDIENTS

SERVES 3-4

Thai Curry Paste

- 1 tablespoon coriander seeds
- 2 cloves
- 4 peppercorns
- 1 inch galangal, peeled and chopped
- 1.5 inch ginger, peeled and chopped
- 2 small green chilis, chopped
- 3 fresh kaffir lime leaves
- ½ cup water
- 2 lemongrass stems, pounded & chopped
- ½ cup fresh basil leaves
- ½ cup fresh coriander leaves

Vegetable Curry

- 1 cup chopped broccoli
- 1 cup chopped zucchini
- 1½ cup bell peppers (red, yellow, green)
- 3 chopped baby corns
- ¼ cup chopped & steamed sweet potato
- 2 cups thick coconut milk
- ½ tablespoon rock salt
- 1 tablespoon jaggery
- 2 tablespoons chopped and roasted peanuts for topping

Brown rice, cooked

PRE-PREPARATION

Prepare thick coconut milk by blending 1 cup coconut with 1 cup water and then straining it.

METHOD

1. Dry roast coriander seeds, cloves and black peppercorns together until coriander seeds turn dark brown.

2. Blend the dry roasted mixture till it turns into a fine powder. In the same blender, add all the remaining ingredients of the thai curry paste (as given in the column on the left), and blend until you get a fine paste.

3. Keep a pot on medium flame and add broccoli, zucchini, bell peppers, baby corn and ½ cup water to it. Let vegetables cook for 15-20 minutes, till they turn soft. After sweet potato is steamed, add it to the pot.

4. Reduce the flame to low and pour the Thai green curry paste and jaggery also to the pot and mix well. Cover the lid for 5 minutes so all flavours come together.

5. Turn off the stove and add coconut milk and salt. Mix well. Close the pot for another 10 minutes. Thai curry is ready.

6. Top it with roasted and chopped peanuts. Serve It with brown rice.

OCCASIONAL

Scan to watch
the video

143

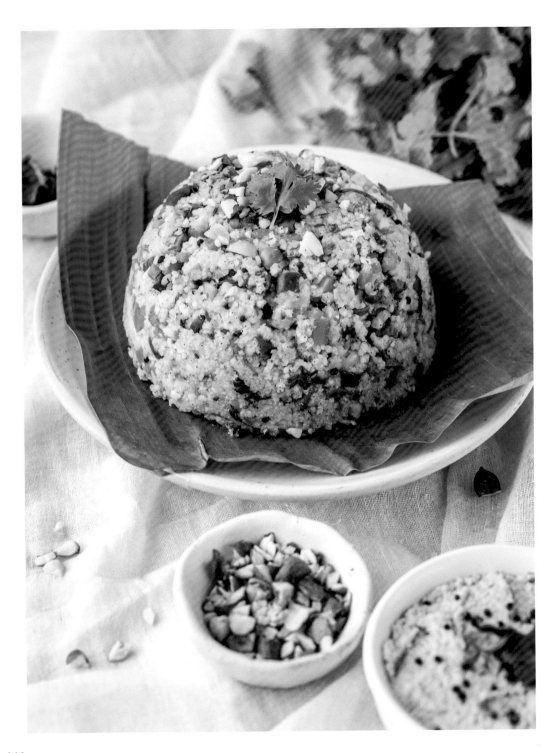

MILLET UPMA

BEST FOR

○ Morning Detox Drink
○ Breakfast

○ Lunch
○ Mid-Meal

○ Dinner
◉ An Occasional Lunch

INGREDIENTS
SERVES 3-4

- 1 cup millet (barnyard, proso or foxtail)
- 3 cups water
- 1 cup green beans, finely chopped
- 1 cup carrot, finely chopped
- 1 cup peas
- ¼ cup coriander, finely chopped

Flavoring

- 2 teaspoons black mustard seeds
- 1 teaspoon cumin seeds
- 2 teaspoons grated fresh ginger
- 2 tablespoons peanuts, chopped
- 15-20 curry leaves
- 2 small green chilis, finely chopped
- ½ teaspoon asafoetida powder
- 2 tablespoons lemon juice
- 2 ½ teaspoon rock salt

Garnish

- ½ tablespoon peanuts, crushed

Coconut Chutney (pg 91)

PRE-PREPARATION

- Soak the millets in water for 2-3 hours.

METHOD

1. Dry roast the mustard seeds, cumin seeds, green chillies, ginger and peanuts in a pot for about 5-8 minutes.
2. Then add curry leaves and roast for another minute.
3. Add beans, carrots & peas to the pot & sauté with roasted spices for 2 minutes.
4. Add 2 cups of water to the pot and cover the lid to let the vegetables cook.
5. After 15 minutes, add the soaked millets and asafoetida with one cup of water to the vegetables and stir. Cover the lid and let the millets cook with vegetables for the flavors to come together. Add more water if needed. Let it cook till there's no more water left in the pot and the millets are cooked with vegetables.
6. Switch off the stove and add lemon, salt & coriander. Stir well. Cover lid for another 2 mins to let the flavors come together.
7. Garnish with roasted peanuts and coriander and serve with coconut chutney.

OCCASIONAL

Scan to watch
the video

145

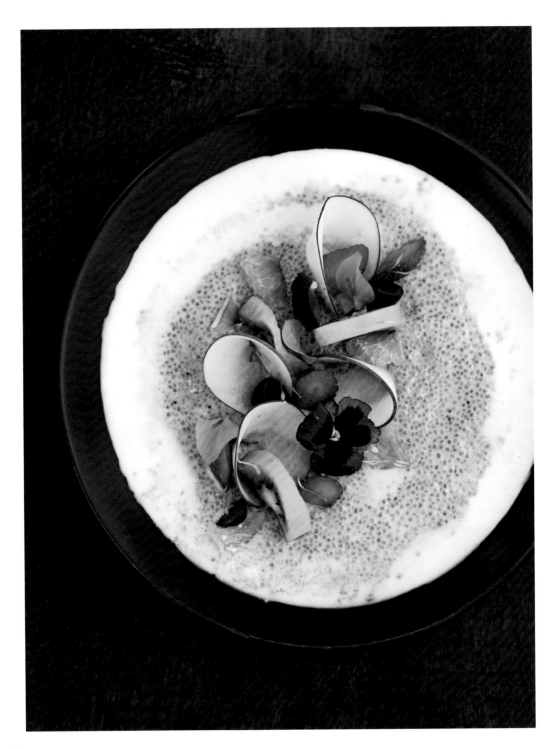

CHIA PUDDING

BEST FOR

○ Morning Detox Drink
○ Breakfast

○ Lunch
○ Mid-Meal

○ Dinner
✓ An Occasional Treat

This pudding is super easy to prepare. Be sure to make this in advance so it has time to thicken up. Chia seeds were the food of the ancient Aztecs. They are great for post-workout. Also, this pudding is fully raw!

INGREDIENTS
SERVES 2-3, MAKES 500 ml

- 1 cup coconut milk
- 1½ tablespoon powdered jaggery
- ½ ripe banana
- ⅛ teaspoon rock salt
- 2 tablespoons chia seeds
- 1 cup chopped mixed fruits (such as banana, mango, grapes, pear, kiwi, orange, pomegranate, berries)

Garnish
- edible flowers (optional)
- fresh seasonal fruits

PRE-PREPARATION
Prepare coconut milk.

METHOD

1. Place coconut milk, jaggery, banana and salt into a blender and blend until smooth.

2. Pour this mixture over chia seeds and let them soak for about 2 hours on the kitchen counter. The chia seeds will swell up and thicken the mixture.

3. Add the chopped fruits to the chia seed mixture. Place the pudding in the refrigerator for 30 minutes before serving, to make it cold.

OCCASIONAL

Scan to watch
the video

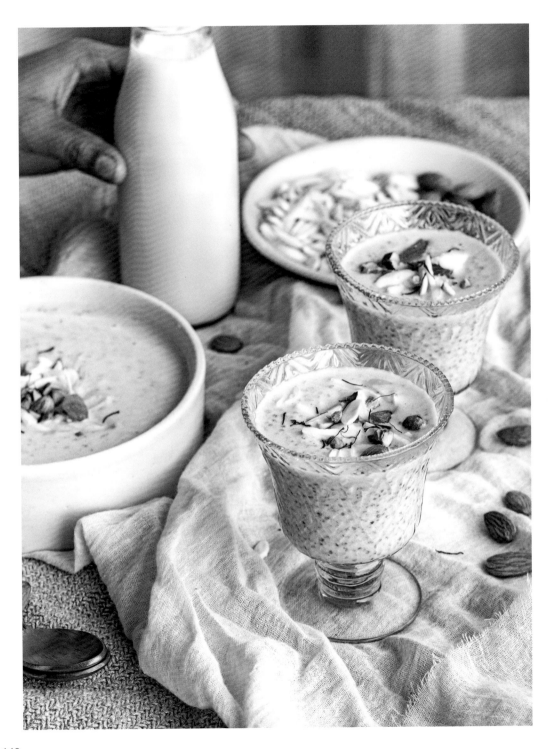

SATVIC KHEER

BEST FOR

○ Morning Detox Drink   ○ Lunch   ○ Dinner
○ Breakfast   ○ Mid-Meal   ✓ An Occasional Treat

Can you imagine eating kheer that is healthy? No sugar, no milk, no ghee, just wholesome ingredients, straight from nature. Instead of fat laden pastries and cookies, serve your guests this healthy dessert. Tell them to guess what it's made of & I promise, they'll be surprised!

INGREDIENTS
SERVES 4-5, MAKES 1 litre

- 1 cup soaked almonds
- ½ cup quinoa
- 3½ cups water
- 6 tablespoons powdered jaggery
- ¼ teaspoon cardamom powder
- 20 strands of saffron (approx.)
- ⅛ teaspoon rock salt

Topping
- 1 tablespoon chopped almonds
- 1 tablespoon chopped pistachios
- 1 tablespoon raisins

PRE-PREPARATION
Soak the almonds in water for about 6 hours. After soaking peel the almonds.

METHOD

1. Place the quinoa in a saucepan with 2 cups of water and bring to a boil. Then, let it simmer for about 45 minutes until the quinoa is fully cooked.

2. Meanwhile, add the peeled almonds and 1½ cups water to a blender and blend until smooth.

3. Add jaggery, cardamom, saffron and salt and blend again.

4. Pour this mixture in a bowl, add the boiled quinoa and stir well. This is your kheer.

5. Place it in a refrigerator for at least 30 minutes. The quinoa will swell up & the kheer will get thick.

6. Top it with almonds, pistachios & raisins and serve.

OCCASIONAL

Scan to watch
the video

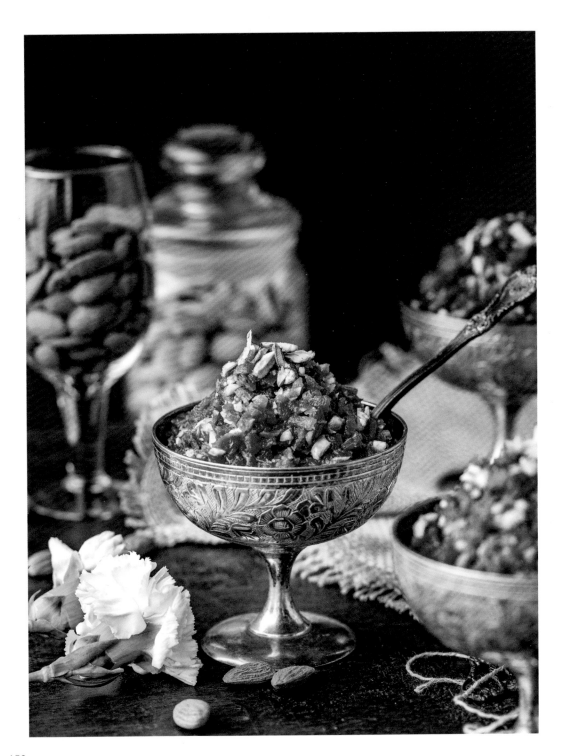

SATVIC GAJAR HALWA

BEST FOR

○ Morning Detox Drink
○ Breakfast

○ Lunch
○ Mid-Meal

○ Dinner
✓ An Occasional Treat

INGREDIENTS
SERVES 6

- 4 cups finely shredded red carrots
- 20 strands of saffron
- ⅓ cup powdered jaggery
- 1 teaspoon green cardamom powder
- ¼ teaspoon rock salt
- 1 teaspoon lemon juice

Thick Coconut Milk
- ½ cup dessicated coconut
- ½ cup water

Date Paste
- ½ cup chopped dates. seedless
- ¼ cup warm water

Topping
- ¼ cup chopped almonds (soaked)
- ¼ cup chopped cashews (soaked)
- 2 tablespoons chopped pistachios

METHOD

1. Place the grated carrots and saffron into a pan and cook on a medium flame for 30 minutes, till the water is absorbed and carrots are soft.

2. Meanwhile, prepare date paste by blending dates and warm water together until smooth.

3. Prepare the thick coconut milk by blending coconut & water together. Sieve the mixture through a nut milk bag / muslin cloth & keep the liquid to be used later.

4. Once carrots have cooked, reduce flame to low. Add jaggery and date paste to the pan and stir together for 30 seconds.

5. Switch off the stove. Add the thick coconut milk, stir & immediately close the lid. Let the coconut milk cook from the heat inside the pan, not directly on flame.

6. Add cardamom, lemon and salt. Stir.

7. Add almonds, cashews and pistachios. Stir.

8. Keep the halwa in the fridge for 30 minutes before serving, so that the flavors can bloom!

- **Tip** Use red carrots to make this halwa. These carrots are available only in winter.

OCCASIONAL

Scan to watch
the video

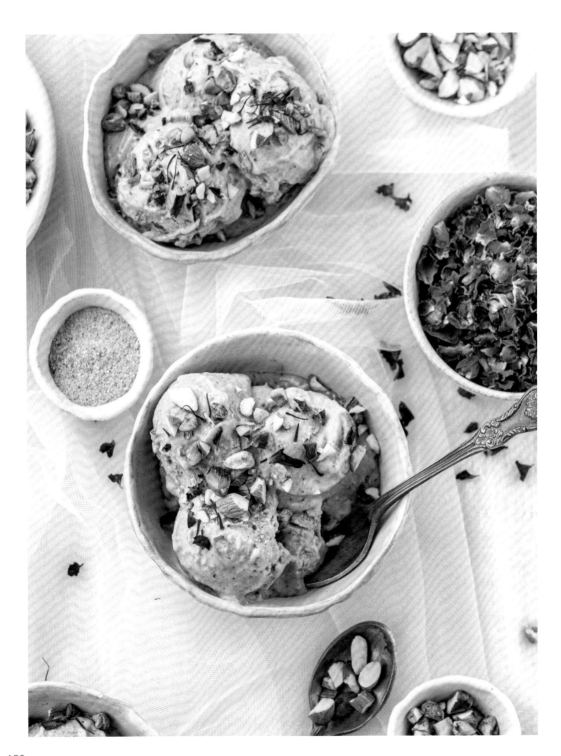

KULFI

BEST FOR

- ○ Morning Detox Drink
- ○ Breakfast
- ○ Lunch
- ○ Mid-Meal
- ○ Dinner
- ✓ An Occasional Treat

Kulfi is a delicious Indian dessert. Many of us think that preparing ice cream at home is a difficult thing to do, but this recipe can be prepared within a few minutes, and you don't even need an ice cream maker for it. The base of this kulfi is made of cashew and coconut.

INGREDIENTS

SERVES 2-3, MAKES 1½ CUPS

Kulfi Ice Cream

- ½ cup soaked cashews
- 1 cup coconut malai
- ¼ cup jaggery, powdered
- 4 dates, seedless
- ⅓ cup coconut water
- 10 strands of saffron
- ⅛ teaspoon green cardamom powder
- ⅛ teaspoon rock salt

Topping

- 1 tablespoon chopped pistachios

PRE-PREPARATION

Soak the cashews in water for about 6 hours.

METHOD

1. Place all the ice cream ingredients in a blender and blend until smooth.

2. Pour the mixture into a shallow glass dish or a steel container, and let it freeze for about 6 hours in the freezer.

3. Before serving, let the ice cream thaw on a counter for 15-30 minutes, until it becomes soft enough to scoop.

4. Top with chopped pistachios and serve.

OCCASIONAL

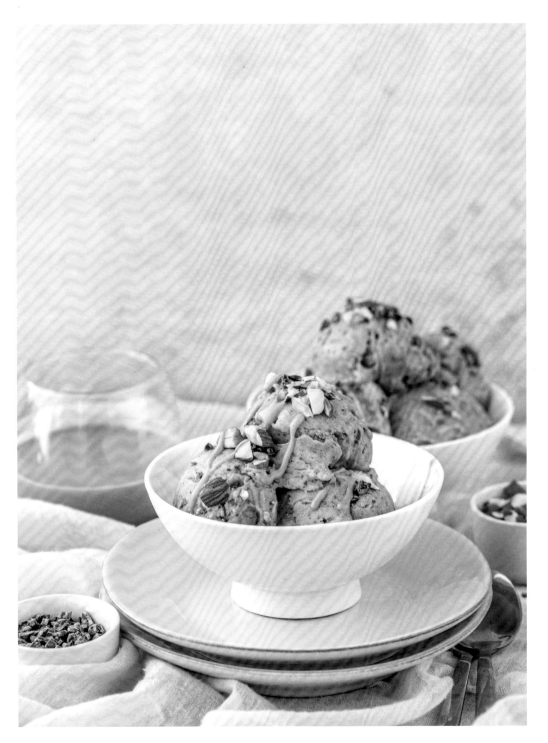

PEANUT BUTTER ICE CREAM

BEST FOR

- ○ Morning Detox Drink
- ○ Breakfast
- ○ Lunch
- ○ Mid-Meal
- ○ Dinner
- ◉ An Occasional Treat

This dessert is ultra creamy, nutty, sweet, and just the right amount of savory. Ask your friends to guess the ingredients and they'll be surprised to know how it's made!

INGREDIENTS

SERVES 3, MAKES 1½ cups

For Making Peanut Butter

- 1 cup peanuts

For Making the Ice Cream

- 6 dates, seedless
- ¼ cup water
- 4 frozen bananas
- 1 tablespoon peanut butter
- ½ tablespoon powdered jaggery
- ⅛ teaspoon rock salt

Topping

- 1 tablespoon almonds, chopped
- 1 tablespoon peanut butter

PRE-PREPARATION

Take the bananas, peel, slice and put in the freezer for about 6 hours.

METHOD

For making peanut butter

1. Heat a pan, add the peanuts and reduce flame to low. Roast peanuts while continuously stirring for 4-5 minutes.

2. Transfer peanuts to a blender and blend for 2-3 minutes, till you get a creamy butter. You will feel it'll never blend, but be patient! The peanuts will first convert into powder and then turn creamy. Do not add any water.

For making peanut butter ice cream

3. Place the dates and water in a blender and blend till a paste is formed.

4. Add the frozen bananas, peanut butter, jaggery and salt to the date paste & blend again until smooth.

5. Scoop out the ice cream into bowls. Top with almonds and peanut butter and serve immediately.

OCCASIONAL

Scan to watch the video

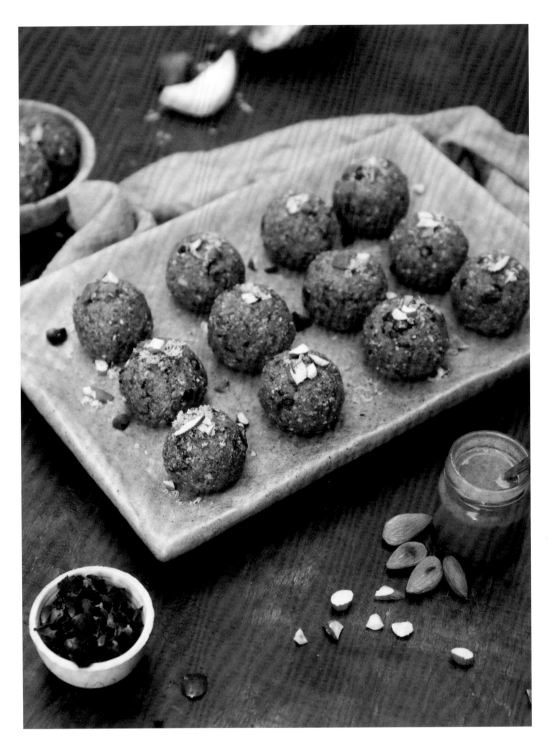

SATVIC LADOO

BEST FOR

◯ Morning Detox Drink   ◯ Lunch   ◯ Dinner

◯ Breakfast   ◯ Mid-Meal   ✅ An Occasional Treat

INGREDIENTS

MAKES 12 LADOOS

- 1 dry coconut (gola)
- 2 tablespoon almond butter*
- 2 tablespoons powdered jaggery
- 2 tablespoons soaked almonds, chopped
- 2 tablespoons dry rose petals

*How to make almond butter?

1. Dry roast almonds in a saucepan over medium flame for 5-7 minutes, stirring in between. Let the almonds cool.
2. Transfer them to a high-speed blender. Blend until creamy, pausing to scrape down the sides as necessary. You will feel it'll never blend, but be patient! The almonds will first convert into powder and then turn creamy. If the mixture gets too hot along the way, stop and let it cool for a few minutes.
3. Transfer it to a jar. Store in the refrigerator for up to 1 week.

METHOD

1. Break the dry coconut into pieces and then shred it finely.
2. Transfer the shredded coconut to a high-speed blender. Blend until creamy, pausing to scrape down the sides as necessary. You will feel it'll never blend, but be patient! The coconut will first convert into powder and then turn soft and buttery. It usually takes 5-7 minutes of blending. If the mixture gets too hot along the way, stop and let it cool for a few minutes.
3. Add this coconut butter to a bowl, along with the almond butter, jaggery, chopped almonds & rose petals. Mix it well using your hands.
4. Shape this batter into small ladoos. Garnish with dry rose petals and serve.

OCCASIONAL

Scan to watch
the video

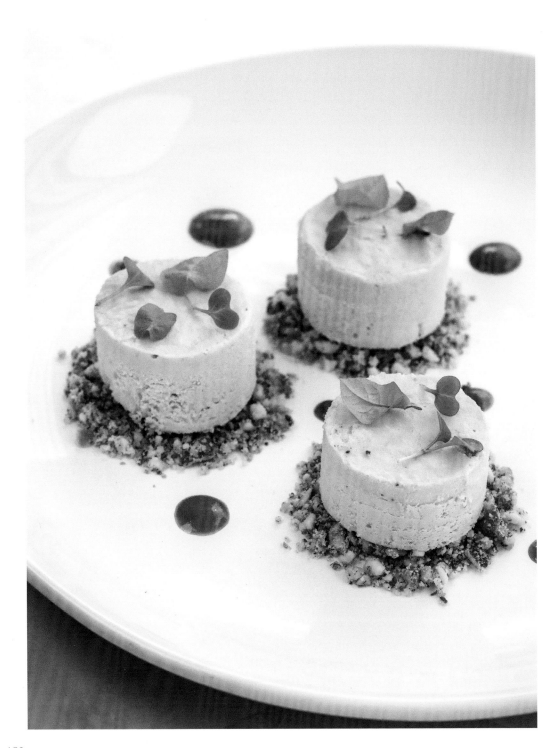

LEMON CHEESECAKE

BEST FOR

○ Morning Detox Drink   ○ Lunch   ○ Dinner
○ Breakfast   ○ Mid-Meal   ✅ An Occasional Treat

One bit of this dessert and you'll never look at cheesecake the same way again. This cheesecake has no dairy, cheese or sugar! But be mindful that it does contain lots of cashews, so must be eaten sparingly.

INGREDIENTS
SERVES 5

Cheesecake
- 1 cup cashews, soaked
- 3 tablespoons powdered jaggery
- ¼ cup water
- 3 tablespoons lemon juice

Lime Gel
- ¼ cup cashews, soaked
- ¼ cup powdered jaggery
- 4 medium leaves of spinach
- ½ tablespoon lemon juice
- ½ tablespoon lemon zest (zest is prepared by finely grating the peel of a fresh lemon)

Ginger Crumble
- ½ cup almonds
- ½ tablespoon jaggery powder
- ¼ teaspoon ginger, grated
- pinch rock salt

Garnish (optional)
- microgreens
- edible flowers

PRE-PREPARATION
Soak the cashews in water for 5-6 hrs.

METHOD

1. To prepare the cheesecake, blend all ingredients in a blender. Pour in a pan. Chill in freezer for 5-6 hours. Once frozen, remove from the pan and cut into squares, circles or triangles. Store in refrigerator until ready to serve.

2. To prepare the lime gel, blend all ingredients until perfectly smooth. Pour in a squeeze bottle and refrigerate.

3. To prepare the ginger crumble, quickly pulse the almonds in a blender. Mix the rest of the ingredients by hand.

4. To assemble all components together, sprinkle 3 piles of ginger crumble on a plate. Place a piece of cheesecake on top of each pile. Garnish with lime gel, microgreens and edible flowers.

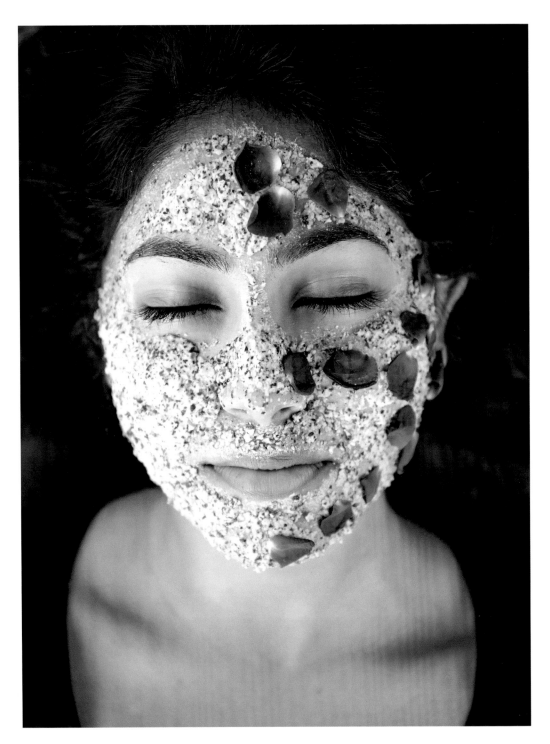

ROSE CLEANSER
FOR FACE & BODY

BEST FOR

 Everyday Use   ○ Occasional Use

Most conventional soaps contain heavy fragrances, nasty parabens, dyes and other chemicals that don't belong on our skin. Our skin is our biggest detox organ so we don't want to coat or clog it with artificial chemicals. This 3-ingredient rose face cleanser is made using 100% natural, and edible ingredients. It takes under 5 minutes to make. It is good for all skin types - dry, oily and sensitive.

INGREDIENTS
MAKES 1 BATCH

- 1 cup oats
- 10 almonds
- ¼ cup dry rose petals

METHOD

1. Blend all the ingredients together until you have a powder. This is your cleanser. Store it in an airtight container for up till 2 weeks.

2. When applying, take a spoonful of the cleanser in a small cup and combine it with some water to form a paste.

3. Rinse your skin with running water. Apply a sufficient amount of the paste to your face or body, massaging in a circular motion for 3-5 minutes to allow the granules to remove dead skin cells.

4. Finally, rinse off well. This makes your skin look and feels refreshed and healthy.

· **Tip** Make sure that the powder in your container does not come in contact with water, or otherwise, it may grow mold.

First published in hardback in India by
Satvic Movement 2018
DLF Phase 1, Gurgaon-122002, India
www.satvicmovement.org

ISBN: 978-93-5493-508-4